# TESTING COMPUTER SYSTEMS FOR FDA/MHRA COMPLIANCE

David Stokes

informa
healthcare

New York London

First published in 2004 by CRC Press LLC.
This edition published in 2010 by Informa Healthcare, Telephone House, 69-77 Paul Street, London EC2A 4LQ, UK.

Simultaneously published in the USA by Informa Healthcare, 52 Vanderbilt Avenue, 7th Floor, New York, NY 10017, USA.

Informa Healthcare is a trading division of Informa UK Ltd. Registered Office: 37–41 Mortimer Street, London W1T 3JH, UK. Registered in England and Wales number 1072954.



A CIP record for this book is available from the British Library.

Library of Congress Cataloging-in-Publication Data available on application

ISBN-13: 9780849321634

Orders may be sent to: Informa Healthcare, Sheepen Place, Colchester, Essex CO3 3LP, UK
Telephone: +44 (0)20 7017 5540
Email: CSDhealthcarebooks@informa.com
Website: http://informahealthcarebooks.com/

For corporate sales please contact: CorporateBooksIHC@informa.com
For foreign rights please contact: RightsIHC@informa.com
For reprint permissions please contact: PermissionsIHC@informa.com

# Table of Contents

## List of Tables



## List of Figures

# Author's Preface

This version of *Testing Computer Systems For FDA/MHRA Compliance* replaces and updates four previous guides that specifically covered the topics of software module, software integration, hardware and system acceptance testing. It consolidates much of the original material on how to test, and includes valuable additional material on why we test, what to test, and how to test. The MHRA (Medicines and Healthcare Products Regulatory Agency) was formerly known as the MCA (Medicines Control Agency) and is based in London.

This version brings together current best practice in computer systems testing in the regulatory environment – specifically the pharmaceutical and related healthcare manufacturing industries. We reference content from the latest GAMP 4 Guide [1] (Package Configuration, the revised software and hardware categories and risk analysis) and show how the principles detailed in GAMP 4 can be used to define a pragmatic approach to testing.

Much of this best testing practice has been established for a number of years, and many of the basic ideas date back to the 1980s (and even earlier). Although the specific regulations vary from industry to industry, the approach and ideas contained in this guideline can certainly be used in other regulated sectors, such as the nuclear and financial industries.

In the two years since publication of the original guidelines the world of information technology (IT) has continued to move forward apace. Despite the bursting of the 'dot.com bubble' some useful tools have emerged from the Internet frenzy and are now available for testing of computer systems.

Most recent developments have been driven by the need to test large Internet based systems, and some manufacturers have invested the time and money to provide automated test tools that can be used in a manner which comply with the stringent requirements of regulations such as 21CFR Part 11 (Electronic Records and Electronic Signatures).

New content is included in this guideline, covering the compliant use of such tools, which will be of specific interest and value to those companies and individuals thinking of investing in such technology.

Additional thought has been given to trying to clarify the relationship and responsibilities of the system 'user' and 'supplier'. This includes where testing starts in the project lifecycle, who does what testing, where the lines of responsibility start and end and the differences in the terminology used in the healthcare and general IT sectors.

We have tried to produce guidance that reflects the renewed approach of the FDA and other regulatory agencies towards systematic inspections and risk-based validation with an underlying scientific rationale. While the acceptability of some of the ideas put forward will no doubt be subject to discussion in many Life Science companies, we hope the guide will prove to be a valuable starting point

*David Stokes*, Spring 2003

# Authors' Preface

[illegible]

CHAPTER 1

# Purpose

The purpose of this guideline is to:

- Demonstrate the value of a systematic approach to computer systems testing ('why we test').
- Provide a pragmatic method of determining the degree of testing necessary for any given system ('what to test').
- Provide a detailed guide to the recommended contents of computer systems test specifications and how to produce these in the most cost effective manner possible.
- Show where computer system testing sits in the full validation life cycle and where the tests sit in relation to the overall project.
- Provide practical advice on how to conduct computer system tests ('how to test').
- Provide guidance on the use of automated test tools in a compliant environment.

CHAPTER 2

# Scope

## 2.1 What This Guideline Covers

This guideline covers the following areas:

i. The cost/benefits of conducting an appropriate degree of system testing.
ii. A practical approach to determining exactly what is 'an appropriate degree of system testing' and how this can be justified (and documented) from a regulatory perspective.
iii. The life cycle management relating to the development of Test Specifications and the conducting of these system tests.
iv. The roles and responsibilities of those involved with the development of Test Specifications and the execution of these system tests.
v. The relationship between System Test Specification(s) and other project documentation.
vi. The relationship between the system tests and other aspects of the project implementation.
vii. Recommended content for inclusion in System Test Specification(s).
viii. A traceability matrix defining how the System Test Specification(s) relate to the System (design) Specification(s).
ix. The selection, implementation and use of compliant automated test tools.
x. References and Appendices, including:
    - A checklist of questions to be used when developing System Test Specification(s)
    - Templates for documenting typical system test results

In this guideline the term System Test Specification(s) refers to any of the following separate Test Specifications defined in GAMP 4:

- Hardware Test Specification
- Software Module Test Specification(s)
- Software Integration Test Specification
- Package Configuration Test Specification(s)
- System Acceptance Test Specification

Further details on the specific purpose and content of such Test Specification(s) is given later in this guideline, as well as other commonly defined testing such as Factory Acceptance Test Specifications, Site Acceptance Test Specifications and so on.

## 2.2 When Is This Guideline Applicable?

This guideline can be used for any project where there is a requirement for system testing and may be used to help test planning, Test Specification development, test execution, test reporting and test management.

### 2.3 Who Is This Guideline Intended For?

This guideline is of value to:

- Those involved with developing Validation Master Plans (VMP) and Validation Plans (VP)
- Those involved with developing Project Quality Plans (PQP)
- Those involved in reviewing and approving Test Specifications
- Those responsible for developing System (Design) Specification(s) (to ensure the 'testability' of the overall software design)
- Those involved with the development and execution of the System Test Specification(s)
- Project Managers whose project scope includes system testing

CHAPTER 3

# Why Do We Test?

There are a number of reasons given in answer to the question 'why do we test?' Some of the answers are more useful than others; it is important that anyone involved in testing understands the basic reason why computer systems are tested.

## 3.1 Because the Regulators Require Us To...

Testing is a fundamental requirement of current best practice with regard to achieving and maintaining regulatory compliance. Although the need to test computer systems is defined by certain regulations and in supporting guidance documents, the way in which computer systems should be tested is not defined in detail.

Although the nature and extent of computer systems testing must be defined and justified on a system by system basis, it is a basic premise that most computer systems will require some degree of testing.

Failure to test will undermine any validation case and the compliant status of the system. Where exposed, during regulatory inspection, this may lead to citations and warning letters being issued and possibly a failure to grant new drug/device licenses, license suspension, products being placed on import restrictions, etc.

Regulatory expectation is based on the premise that computer systems be tested in order to confirm that user and functional requirements have been met and in order to assure data integrity. These, in turn, are driven by a regulatory need to assure patient safety and health.

## 3.2 Because the Quality Assurance Department Requires Us To...

The role of the Quality Assurance (QA) department (Department of Regulatory Affairs, Compliance and Validation department, etc.) in many organisations is a proactive and supportive one. In such organisations the QA department will provide independent assurance that regulations are met and will help to define policies outlining the need for, and approach to, testing.

However, in some companies this may lead to a situation where the QA department becomes responsible for policing the validation of computer systems and often defines the need to test computer systems within an organisation. The danger here is that testing is conducted purely 'because the QA department requires it' – other reasons for testing are not understood.

This QA role is defined at a corporate level and those organisations where the IT and Information Systems (IS) departments and QA work hand-in-hand usually conduct the most appropriate and pragmatic level of testing.

This is not always the case. In some organisations, one standard of testing may be inappropriately applied to all systems, simply because this has always been the approach in the past. It is important that computer systems validation policies state and explain the need for testing, rather than mandate an approach that must be followed, regardless of the system under test.

### 3.3 Because We've Always Done It This Way...

In many organisations there is a single standard or level of testing mandated for all.

However, one standard cannot be appropriately applied to systems that may range in scope from a global Enterprise Resource Planning (ERP) system to a small spreadsheet. In this guideline the term system covers all such systems including embedded systems. A scaleable, cost effective and risk-based approach must therefore be taken, as defined in Section 4.1.

### 3.4 Because It Saves Money!

So far, the only justifiable requirement for testing is based upon meeting regulatory expectation; if this were the only reason, industries not required to meet regulatory requirements would possibly not test systems at all. There is, however, an overriding reason for testing computer systems.

This primary reason for testing systems is that it is more cost effective to 'go live' with systems that are known to function correctly. Regulatory expectations are therefore fully in-line with business benefits.

Most people involved with projects where there has been insufficient testing know that those problems only exposed after 'go live' will be the most time consuming and most expensive to correct.

In many Life Science organisations there is political pressure to implement systems in unrealistic timescales and at the lowest possible capital cost. This often leads to a culture where testing is minimised in order to reduce project timescales and implementation costs.

Although this may often succeed in delivering a system, the real effect is to:

- Reduce the effectiveness and efficiency of the system at 'go live'.
- Increase the maintenance and support costs.
- Require a costly programme of corrective actions to be implemented, to correct faults and meet the original requirements.
- At worst, roll out a system which does not meet the basic user requirements.

The net effect is to increase the overall cost of implementing the system (although this may be hidden on an operational or support budget) and to delay, or prevent the effective and efficient use of the system.

When a system is appropriately tested it is more likely to operate correctly from 'go-live'. This improves user confidence and improves overall acceptance of the system (it is no coincidence that system or user acceptance testing is an important part of the test process). The system will operate more reliably and will cost less to maintain and support.

Senior management and project sponsors need to understand that testing is not an unnecessary burden imposed by the regulators or internal QA departments. Proper testing of the system will ensure that any potential risk to patient safety is minimised; one of the main business justifications is that it will save time and money.

CHAPTER 4

# What to Test

Having stated that a 'one-size-fits-all' approach to system testing is no longer appropriate, the challenge is to define a justifiable approach to testing; to minimise the time and cost of testing, while still meeting regulatory expectations.

This comes down to the basic (and age-old) questions of:

- How much testing to conduct?
- What should be tested for?

Some systems are extremely complex and the concern of the regulatory agencies is that there are almost infinite numbers of paths through the software. This stems from a concern that, unless all paths through the software are tested, how can patient safety be assured under all circumstances?

In large or complex systems it is practically impossible to test each path, but the reasoning for not testing certain paths, options or functions is often made on an arbitrary basis. What is needed is an approach that will allow testing to focus on areas of highest potential risk, but to do so in a justifiable and documented manner

## 4.1 GxP Priority

Appendix M3 in GAMP 4 defines a methodology for determining the GxP Priority of a system. More usefully, this approach can be used to determine the GxP Priority of specific functions in a large or complex system.

In order to determine a sensible approach to testing a system it is useful to determine the GxP Priority of the system or the GxP Priority of different parts (functions) of the system. This can then be used in justifying the approach to testing. Different component parts of the system may be more GxP critical than others, for example, Quality versus Financial functions. Assessing the GxP criticality of each function allows testing to be focused on the areas of greatest risk. There are other risks, which may need to be considered and these are discussed in Appendix F.

## 4.2 Software/Hardware Category

Appendix M4 in GAMP 4 defines categories of software and hardware.

With the exception of some embedded systems, most systems will be made up of software of different categories. For instance, a system may consist of an Operating System (software category 1) and a configurable application (software category 4).

Most systems will be based upon standard hardware (hardware category 1), although some systems may be based upon custom hardware (hardware category 2).

Once the component parts of a system have been categorised they can be used to help determine a justifiable approach to cost effective testing.

### 4.3 Test Rationale and Test Policies

Based upon a combination of the GxP criticality of a system or function, and the software and/or hardware category of a system or function, it is possible to define a consistent and justifiable approach to system testing.

Based upon the GAMP 4 GxP Priority and the software/hardware category of the system, a consistent approach to testing can be documented. This may be in the form of a Test Strategy Matrix and defined Test Approaches, examples of which are given below. There are also other risk factors that should be borne in mind, and these are discussed in Appendix F.

Note that the examples shown are provided as a case-in-point only. An organisation may wish to define their own corporate Testing Policy and a standard Test Strategy Matrix and Test Approaches, based upon the principles given below. Other approaches and notation may be defined (in the examples below 'S' refers to software testing, 'H' to hardware testing and 'F' to Functional Testing).

Once an organisation has agreed upon standard approaches to risk-based testing, they can be used as the basis for defining system specific Test Strategy Matrices and Test Approaches for the testing of individual systems.

Table 4.1 and Table 4.2 show how GxP Criticality and software/hardware category can be cross-referenced to a test approach.

**Table 4.1 – Example of Software Testing Criticality**

| | | *GAMP 4 GxP Criticality* | | |
|---|---|---|---|---|
| | | *Low* | *Medium* | *High* |
| GAMP 4 | 1 * | Test Approach F | Test Approach F | Test Approach F |
| Software | 2 | Test Approach F | Test Approach F | Test Approach S1 |
| Category | 3 | Test Approach F | Test Approach F | Test Approach S1 |
| | 4 | Test Approach F | Test Approach S2 | Test Approach S3 |
| | 5 | Test Approach S4 | Test Approach S5 | Test Approach S6 |

* No testing of Category 1 (Operating System) is required – this is tested *in situ* with the application it is supporting.

**Table 4.2 – Example of Hardware Testing Criticality**

| | | *GAMP 4 GxP Criticality* | | |
|---|---|---|---|---|
| | | *Low* | *Medium* | *High* |
| GAMP 4 | 1 * | Test Approach F | Test Approach F | Test Approach F |
| Hardware Category | 2 | Test Approach H1 | Test Approach H2 | Test Approach H3 |

* No testing of Category 1 (standard hardware components) is required – this is implicitly tested by the integration testing of the system.

Table 4.3 describes the testing and review required for each of the Test Approaches defined.

**Table 4.3 – Example of Test Approaches based upon Software or Hardware Criticality**

| *Test Approach* | *Description* |
|---|---|
| F | No specific hardware or software testing is required.<br>Hardware and software will be tested as part of overall System Acceptance Testing (Functional Testing). |
| S1 | Software will be tested as part of overall System Acceptance Testing (Functional Testing).<br>Testing outside standard operating ranges is required in order to predict failure modes.<br>100% of System Acceptance Test Specifications and Results are subject to Quality function review and approval. |
| S2 | In additional to System Acceptance (Functional) Testing, software must be subject to stress testing during normal operating conditions to challenge:<br>– Basic system (log-in) access<br>– User (role) specific functional access<br>– System administration access<br>– Network security<br>All Test Specifications and Results are subject to peer review.<br>50% of Package Configuration Test Specifications and 50% of related Results are subject to independent Quality function review and approval.<br>100% of all System Acceptance Test Specifications and Results are subject to independent Quality function review and approval. |
| S3 | In addition to System Acceptance (Functional) Testing, software must be subject to comprehensive stress testing across normal and abnormal operating conditions in order to challenge:<br>– Basic system (log-in) access<br>– User (role) specific functional access<br>– System administration access<br>– Network security<br>All Test Specifications and Results are subject to peer review.<br>100% of Package Configuration Test Specifications and 100% of related Results are subject to independent Quality function review.<br>100% of all System Acceptance Test Specifications and Results are subject to independent Quality function review. |
| S4 | Software Module Testing is mandated prior to System Integration Tests and System Acceptance Testing.<br>Testing is required only within standard operating range.<br>All Test Specifications and Results are subject to peer review.<br>25% of Software Module Test Specifications and 10% of all Software Module Test Results are subject to independent Quality function review.<br>25% of all Software Integration Specification and related test Results are subject to independent Quality function review.<br>100% of all System Acceptance Test Specifications and Results are subject to independent Quality function review. |
| S5 | Software Module Testing mandated prior to System Integration Tests and System Acceptance Testing.<br>Testing only within standard operating range required for Software Module Tests.<br>Testing outside standard operating range required for Software Integration Tests in order to predict failure modes.<br>All Test Specifications and Results are subject to peer review.<br>50% of Software Module Test Specifications and 50% of all Software Module Test Results are subject to independent Quality function review.<br>50% of all Software Integration Specification and related test Results are subject to independent Quality function review.<br>100% of all System Acceptance Test Specifications and Results are subject to independent Quality function review. |

| *Test Approach* | *Description* |
|---|---|
| S6 | Software Module Testing mandated prior to System Integration Tests and System Acceptance Testing.<br>Testing only within standard operating range required for Software Module Tests.<br>Testing outside standard operating range required for Software Integration Tests in order to predict failure modes.<br>All Test Specifications and Results are subject to peer review.<br>100% of Software Module Test Specifications and 100% of all Software Module Test Results are subject to independent Quality function review.<br>25% of all Software Integration Specification and related test Results are subject to independent Quality function review.<br>100% of all System Acceptance Test Specifications and Results are subject to independent Quality function review. |
| H1 | No hardware specific testing required. Will be tested as part of overall System Acceptance Testing (Functional Testing)<br>100% of all System Acceptance Test Specifications and Results are subject to independent Quality function review. |
| H2 | Hardware assembled from custom components procured from single supplier requires hardware integration tests to be performed to test adequate performance across all normal operating ranges. May be conducted by supplier so long as acceptable documentary proof is provided.<br>Hardware assembled from custom components procured from multiple suppliers requires hardware integration tests to be performed to test adequate performance across all normal operating ranges.<br>All Test Specifications and Results are subject to peer review. |
| H2 | 50% of all Hardware Test Specification(s) and related test Results subject to independent Quality function review.<br>100% of all System Acceptance Test Specifications and Results are subject to independent Quality function review. |
| H3 | Hardware assembled from custom components procured from single supplier requires hardware integration tests to be performed to test adequate performance across all normal operating ranges. Should be witnessed by user representative if conducted by supplier.<br>Hardware assembled from custom components procured from multiple suppliers requires hardware integration tests to be performed to test adequate performance across all normal operating ranges. Also requires hardware integration tests to be performed outside normal operating ranges in order to predict failure modes.<br>100% of all Hardware Test Specification(s) and related test Results subject to independent Quality function review.<br>100% of all System Acceptance Test Specifications and Results are subject to independent Quality function review. |

Such an approach may be used to justify the nature and level of both testing and review to be applied to any individual system, or to the specific parts (functions) of a complex system.

However, the move away from full (100%) review of test specifications and test results by an independent QA function needs to be justified within any organisation. For this to be accepted as a risk-based approach to testing (validation), based upon a justifiable and rigorous scientific approach, it is important to have proof that the integrity or quality of the testing process is not compromised.

This can best be obtained by monitoring long-term trends in the testing process, and will almost certainly require the QA department to monitor the efficacy and integrity of the peer review process, with subsequent traceable changes to the testing policy. This can be achieved by comparing test statistics taken during the testing process and by sampling and reviewing a random selection of test specifications and results subjected to a peer review process. As with any sampling, there must be a scientific rationale for the sample size taken.

If the peer review process adversely impacts upon the quality or integrity of the testing process, corrective actions must be taken. This may include further training for those involved in testing, or the creation of a dedicated test team. If this does not improve the situation, the policy may need to increase the level of QA review and approval, until such a time as acceptable standards of peer review are achieved. When defining such an approach in a test policy, the following key points must be borne in mind:

- The method and rationale for revising the test policy and test approaches must be explained, including the basis for any sampling.
- It is better to start with a closely monitored peer review process and relax the QA review over time, rather than initially remove all QA reviews and tighten up again at a later date.
- Such a test policy can never mandate the scope, nature and level of testing for any specific system. The policy should seek to provide consistent guidance and also identify circumstances where a more thorough testing approach may be appropriate.

Note: more complex risk-based criteria can also be used to allocate different software modules to appropriate testing approaches (see Appendix F – Risk-Based Testing).

## 4.4 Testing or Verification

The terms ***testing*** and ***verification*** are often used when validating a system and the two are often (incorrectly) used interchangeably. Testing is different from verification and there should be clarity as to which parts of a system are to be subject to testing and which parts will be verified.

In simple terms, components that can be subjected to a repeatable set of input criteria, which will produce a predictable and repeatable set of output criteria (results), ***can be tested***. This means that a test script can be written which defines both input criteria and expected output criteria, and upon which the actual output criteria (results) may be recorded.

It may not be possible or practical to subject other components of the system to input criteria, or it may be difficult to observe the resultant output criteria. In these cases it may be possible to ***verify*** the correct operation of the system or component by other means.

As an example, consider a set of data being imported from a legacy system (about to be decommissioned) into a replacement system.

Data migration from the old system to the new system will possibly involve data (format) conversion, data export, data cleansing, data import and final data conversion. Software routines can be written to perform all of these functions, but must be tested to ensure that they work in a predictable and repeatable manner across a wide range of datasets. These tests should include the use of out-of-range data, corrupted data and 'illegal' data formats. This ensures that the results of routines can be predicted and assured for all datasets that are to be migrated and that any errors will be trapped and flagged.

Where a large number of complex datasets are to be converted, it is obviously cost effective to develop and test such routines. This may not be cost-justified when there is only a single dataset, which contains just 16 floating-point numbers.

In certain cases it will be more cost effective to verify the data in the new system. In the simple case quoted above, this may involve a simple data import (entering the data directly into the new system), and manually checking data in the new system against the data in the old system (either on-screen or as hard copy). For data classified as medium or high GxP criticality, this may be subject to independent checking by a second person. This manual process would not test the data transport mechanism but would ***verify*** the results of the process.

In a similar way, other parts of a system build cannot be tested, but must be verified by manual inspection. Examples of this may include:

- Checking the version of an installed operating system.
- Checking the serial numbers of hardware components installed within a system.

When considering what to test, it should be appreciated that, when it is impossible ***to test*** some items, they must still ***be verified***. Where testing is possible, but verification is the chosen route (for reasons of cost effectiveness or efficiency), this should be justified as part of the test strategy.

CHAPTER 5

# The Test Strategy

Any approach to testing must be documented in order to demonstrate that an appropriate risk-based approach has been taken.

For small or simple systems the test strategy may be obvious at the start of the project. Where it is possible to reference a corporate (division or site) policy, this may be included in the Validation Master Plan (VMP), or possibly in the Project Quality Plan (PQP).

For larger or more complex systems it is useful to define a test strategy in a separate document. This may be either a specific test strategy document, or a high-level qualification protocol document. For very large or complex systems, multiple test strategy documents may be produced, one for each level of testing in addition to an overall summary describing the relationship between the various types of testing and associated test strategies.

For the purposes of this guide, the term 'test strategy' refers to the testing rationale and justification, whether this is included in the VMP, PQP, a separate document, or the installation qualification (IQ), operational qualification (OQ), and performance qualification (PQ) protocols.

Test strategies should include the following sections (where applicable).

## 5.1 Risk-Based Rationale

The approach taken to testing should be based on risk and should be included as part of the test strategy. This includes GxP Priority (see Section 4.1) as well as other risks (see Appendix F – Risk-Based Testing).

## 5.2 The Relationship between Test Specification(s)

Depending upon the complexity and size of the system, different test specifications will be needed. As we have seen above, GAMP 4 defines five types of test specification, namely:

- Hardware Test Specification
- Software Module Test Specification(s)
- Software Integration Test Specification
- Package Configuration Test Specification(s)
- System Acceptance Test Specification

Further specific information on each of these types of testing is given in Appendices 1 to 5. Which of these types of test are needed depends upon the nature of the system (GxP Criticality, software category and hardware category).

Guidance on which of these tests is required can be defined in a test strategy. GAMP 4 includes these types of testing in both the Documentation in the Life Cycle Model (Figure 8.1

in GAMP 4) and the Standalone Systems Lifecycle Activities and Documentation Model (Figure 9.3 in GAMP 4).

Extracting the test specific documentation and activities from these models produces the following diagram, which clearly shows the relationship between the various test specification(s) and test activities.

The order in which these are shown should never be varied. The sequencing of the various test activities should be defined as prerequisites in the test strategy. In summary these are:

- All test specification(s) must be approved before the corresponding test activities commence.
- Any software module testing should be completed prior to the software integration tests commencing. It should be noted that in large systems some parallel testing will take place. As an example, integration testing may commence before all module testing is complete. It is recommended that this is limited to informal testing; formal integration testing is not performed until all software module testing is complete.
- All hardware acceptance tests, package configuration verification, software module and software integration testing must be complete, and signed off, prior to system acceptance testing commencing.

### 5.3 Integrating or Omitting the System Test Specification(s)

Not all of these system test specifications will be needed for every system; some are optional, depending upon the nature of the system being tested. For instance, if a new application is being installed on an existing server, no hardware testing will be required. If there is no bespoke (customised) software, no software module testing will be required. In the case of small or simple systems, all the testing may be defined in a single test specification, which may include elements of all hardware and software testing.

Where test specifications are omitted or integrated the reasons for this should be clearly documented and the rationale justified in the test strategy.

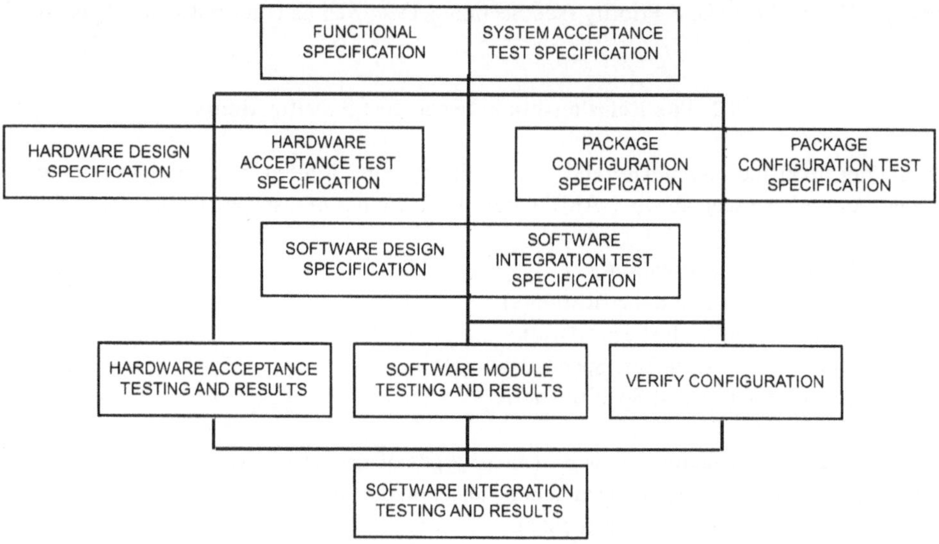


**Figure 5.1 – The Relationship between Test Specifications and Test Activities.**

### 5.3.1 Hardware Acceptance Test Specification and Testing

Hardware acceptance tests are only generally required for customised hardware (Hardware Category 2). Where the system is based upon standard hardware in widespread use, hardware specific acceptance testing is usually not required (although testing of connected hardware components may be required). See Appendix A for further details

### 5.3.2 Package Configuration Test Specification and Testing

Certain types of system require configuration (the setting of various software parameters that determine how the package functions) rather than programming. Typical examples of such systems are Enterprise Resource Planning (ERP) systems and Laboratory Information Systems (LIMS). Some systems combine a degree of configuration with traditional programming (coding).

Any system that includes any degree of configuration setting should have a package configuration specification and should be subjected to site acceptance testing (SAT) as a minimum. For highly configurable systems, it is useful to verify the correct configuration of the system prior to the SAT. It may also be possible to perform a lower level of package configuration testing prior to the full SAT (see Appendix B for details).

### 5.3.3 Software Module Test Specification and Testing

Software module testing is normally required where customised or bespoke software modules have been developed as part of the system or application (GAMP software category 5). This may include customised components of systems that generally consist of category 3 or 4 software.

Where the system or application does not include customised software (lines of code, ladder logic, etc.) then the software module test specification or testing may be omitted (see Appendix C for further details).

### 5.3.4 Software Integration Test Specification and Testing

Systems constructed from multiple bespoke modules, or multiple standard software components or packages, require a software integration test specification; thus providing adequate proof that the various modules/components integrate in an acceptable manner, and that integration is robust and functional.

Systems that consist solely of software categories 1, 2, 3 or 4 may require little or no software module integration testing, so long as the component packages have a proven track record in the Life Sciences market place. In this case the software integration test specification or testing may be omitted. Package integration testing may still be required if individual software packages have not been used in combination before.

If any of these packages have been modified (and is therefore treated as software category 5), or if an unproven package is integrated as part of the overall solution, software integration testing is required (see Appendix D for further details).

### 5.3.5 System Acceptance Test Specification and Testing

For simple or small systems, a separate phase of system acceptance testing may not be required. This will normally be the case for systems comprised solely of software category 1, 2 and possibly category 3 software. This is usually justified when the equipment or system is in widespread use in the Life Science industries and is known to meet the defined business (user) and functional requirements. Although some form of acceptance testing against user requirements will still be required, a separate system acceptance test specification or phase of testing may be omitted (see Appendix E for further details).

### 5.3.6 Integrating Test Specifications and Testing

In the case of small or simple systems, it is not cost effective or justifiable to produce separate test specifications for each type of test. The various types of testing may be combined in a lesser number of test specification documents, possibly combining the recommended content for each type. In very small or very simple systems all levels of testing may be combined into a single test specification.

Consolidation of test specifications is especially useful in the case of embedded systems, where it may be difficult to separate software testing from hardware testing (and possibly electrical and/or pneumatic testing etc.).

## 5.4 The Role of Factory and Site Acceptance Tests

Depending upon the scope of the project, Hardware Acceptance Testing, Software Module Testing, Package Configuration Testing, Software Integration Testing and some System Acceptance Testing may be performed at the supplier's premises known as factory acceptance testing (FAT), or on site, known as site acceptance testing (SAT).

Many suppliers use the terms FAT and SAT to describe the standard testing they perform on their systems or equipment and this is more common with suppliers to a broader range of industries than just the Life Science industries. These are often contractual milestones, on which a stage payment may be based (assuming successful completion). The following paragraphs are provided to help explain how these tests may be leveraged to reduce the scope of any additional (or duplicate) testing.

Usually the system will not be deemed as having been subject to system acceptance testing until at least some of these tests have been performed *in situ*/on site. This is because the Functional Testing of some system features can only be performed when the system is properly installed in its final environment, with all interfaces and support infrastructure in place.

FATs are usually preceded by formal development testing — this is part of the supplier's software development life cycle/quality management system. Formal client testing may commence with the factory acceptance test, but additional site acceptance testing is useful to ensure that:

- The system actually delivered to site is the system that was tested in the factory (by checking hardware serial numbers, software version numbers, ID tags, etc.).
- The system has suffered no damage during shipment that would adversely affect the functional performance of the system.
- System functions that can only be properly tested *in situ* can be performed.

Although unusual, it may be possible or necessary to omit any separate factory acceptance testing and perform the full system acceptance test on site, as part of a site acceptance test. From a project perspective this is not desirable, since testing on site is usually more time consuming and more costly than factory testing. From a financial perspective, as much of the testing as is practical should be performed as part of the standard factory acceptance test.

If appropriate, the System Acceptance Test Specification may be split into two parts, one covering the Factory Acceptance Tests and one covering the Site Acceptance Tests.

Where both Factory Acceptance Testing and Site Acceptance Testing are performed, these will have a relationship with the IQ and OQ as follows:

- Factory Acceptance Testing will be performed first, executing as much of testing as is practical.
- The system will be shipped to the site and the Installation Qualification will be performed. This usually relates to the system hardware (and possibly the firmware, operating system and database software — see Appendix A).
- Site Acceptance Test will then be performed, executing the remaining content of the System Acceptance Testing.
- Operational Qualification will then be performed.

### 5.4.1 The Relationship between IQ, OQ and FATs and SATs

It should be noted that the Site Acceptance Testing and the Operation Qualification Testing largely fulfil the same objectives (testing against the Functional Specification) and that these may usefully be performed at the same time or combined.

Note that decisions on the need for Factory and Site Acceptance Testing, the timing of these with the respect to the IQ and OQ and the possible combination of these may be taken in the early stages of the project. This decision should be documented as part of the Validation Master Plan or in the Project Quality Plan. If this is not the case, the relationship between Factory Acceptance Testing and Site Acceptance Testing should be documented in the Test Strategy.

Wherever possible it is desirable to reference the Supplier's standard testing. Formal IQ and OQ Reports may reference the Supplier's standard testing, which may be conducted as part of standard Factory or Site Acceptance Testing. This may significantly reduce the scope of additional or duplicate user testing and assumes that the level of documented evidence is sufficient to support the validation case, which is in turn dependant upon the GxP criticality of the system (risk).

The relationship between the various Design Specifications, Test Specifications, FATs and SATs is shown in the following diagram (Figure 5.2).

Figure 5.2 shows that:

- The development of Test Specifications takes place at the same time as the correspondent Design Specification (this is of course done by a separate team). This reduces the project implementation time scales and helps ensure that the Functional and Design Specifications are testable.
- Hardware Acceptance Testing is more likely to take place as part of the FAT, but some elements of hardware testing may only be completed *in situ*, on site, during the SAT.
- Software Module Testing and Package Configuration Testing are more likely to take place as part of the FAT but some may only be completed on site during the SAT.
- Software Integration Testing starts during the FAT, but some of this can only be conducted on site during the SAT.
- The results of the Hardware and Software Module Testing can all be referenced or summarised as part of the Installation Qualification.
- The results of the Package Configuration and Software Integration Testing can all be referenced or summarised as part of the Operational Qualification.
- Some System Acceptance Testing may be conducted as part of the FAT, but many Acceptance Tests can only be conducted as part of the SAT.

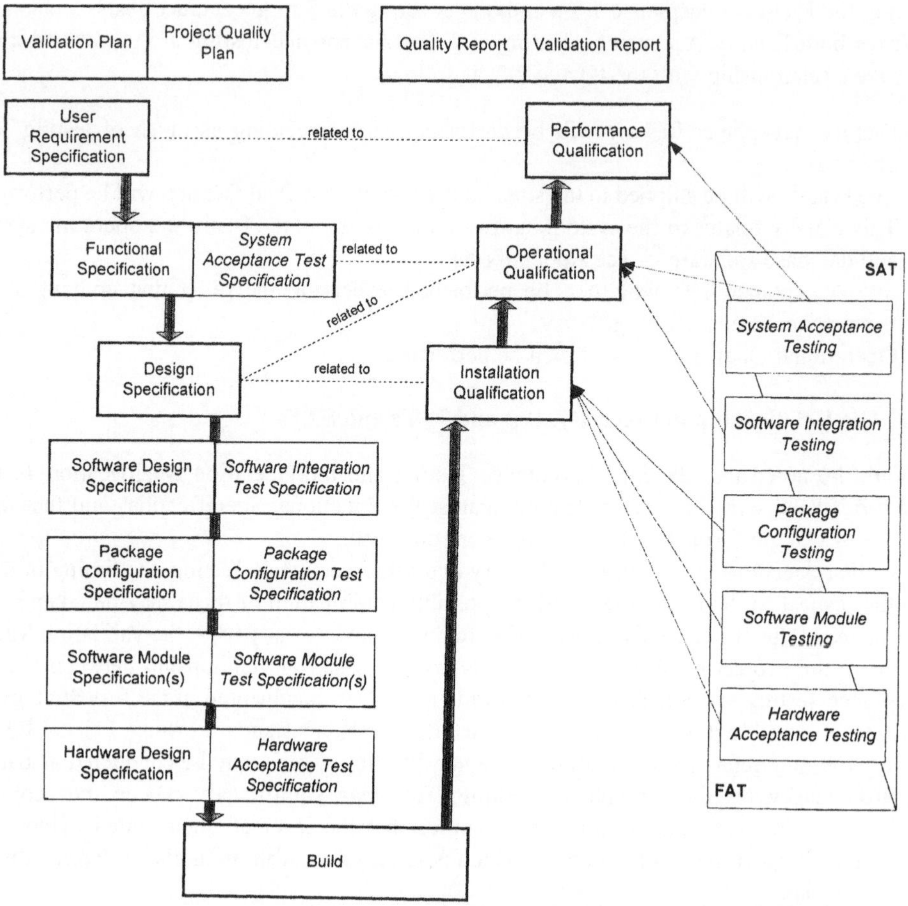


**Figure 5.2 – Relationship between Design Specifications, Test Specifications, FATs, SATs and IQ, OQ and PQ.**

- The results of the System Acceptance Testing can be referenced or summarised as part of the Operation Qualification or Performance Qualification, depending upon the exact nature of the tests concerned.

Note that these interrelationships are summarised in a traceability matrix in Appendix G – Traceability Matrices.

## 5.5 Roles and Responsibilities

The usual roles and responsibilities associated with the preparation of the System Test Specifications and the conducting of the associated tests should be defined in the Test Strategy, as listed below. Note however, that these roles and responsibilities may be changed or shared, according to the specific requirements of a project.

Specifically, the role of supplier may be fulfilled by a user internal function such as IT, Information Systems, Internal Support or an Engineering group.

In addition, the contractual relationship and/or a good long term working relationship may allow the supplier to assume more of the responsibilities usually associated with the role of the user.

There is also an opposite to this situation, where there is a new working relationship, or where the Validation Plan requires the user to put additional validation activities in place in make up for deficiencies in the supplier's quality system. In this case the user may perform more of the supplier's traditional role, or it may require that the user conduct more tests than would usually be the case.

The key roles and responsibilities are usually assigned as summarised in Table 5.1 and in the corresponding explanatory text.

**Table 5.1 – Summary of Testing Roles and Responsibilities**

| | *Supplier* | | | *User* | | | | |
|---|---|---|---|---|---|---|---|---|
| | *QA* | *IS/IT* | *Test Team* | *PM* | *Validation* | *IS/IT* | *Project Team* | *PM* |
| Develop Test Policy | | | | | √ | | | |
| Develop VMP (VP) | | | | | | | √ | |
| Review and Approve VMP (VP) | | | | | √ | | | √ |
| Develop PQP | | | √ | | √ | | | |
| Review and Approve PQP | √ | | | √ | | | | |
| Develop and Review Test Strategy | | | √ | | | | √ | |
| Approve Test Strategy | √ | | | | √ | | | |
| Develop Test Spec's | | | √ | | | | √ | |
| Review Test Spec's | | | √ | | | | √ | |
| Approve Test Spec's | √ | | | | √ | | | |
| Prepare for Tests | | √ | √ | | | √ | √ | |
| Conduct Tests | | | √ | | | | √ | |
| Support Tests | | √ | | | | √ | | |
| Monitor Tests | √ | | | | √ | | | |
| Review and Approve Test Results | √ | | √ | √ | √ | √ | | √ |

### 5.5.1 Supplier

It is the responsibility of the supplier to:

- Develop the Project Quality Plan that identifies the need for supplier specific testing.
- Develop the Hardware Test Specification (if appropriate).
- Develop the Software Module Test Specification (if appropriate).
- Develop the Software Integration Test Specification (if appropriate).
- Develop the Package Configuration Test Specification (if appropriate).
- Develop the System Acceptance Test Specification (if appropriate).
- Physically prepare for the actual tests.
- Conduct the appropriate tests (including recording the results and any retesting as required).

### 5.5.2 User

It is the responsibility of the user to:

- Define the need for the various System Test Specification(s) (usually in the Validation Plan).
- Physically prepare for those tests that will be performed on site.
- Assist with those System Acceptance Tests that will be performed on site.
- Witness the System Acceptance Tests (and any others that may need to be witnessed).

This may be no more that identifying that the System Test Specification(s) are a deliverable of the supplier and the user may choose to delegate all further responsibility to the supplier. This may be acceptable in the case of a reputable supplier with whom the user has worked before.

The System Acceptance Tests are the first major test of overall functionality of the system and it is usual for the user to witness the System Acceptance Tests in order to verify that the system to be supplied meets the agreed Functional Specification.

Where a user chooses not to witness some or all of the System Acceptance Tests the following may suffice as an acceptable alternative:

- Review and/or approve the final System Acceptance Test Specification prior to the System Acceptance Tests commencing.
- Review the results of the System Acceptance Tests and associated documentation as part of the Operational Qualification.

Where the supplier audit has revealed deficiencies in the supplier's testing regime the user may choose to review/approve other Test Specifications and/or witness additional tests (either at the premises of the supplier or on site). These may include the Software Module Tests, the Software Integration Tests, the Package Configuration Tests or the Hardware Tests.

### 5.5.3 Supplier Quality Assurance

It is the role of the supplier's Quality Assurance function to ensure that:

- The System Test Specification(s) are written in accordance with the Project Quality Plan.
- The System Test Specification(s) are approved (by the supplier and, if required, the user) prior to the corresponding level of System Testing commencing.
- The System Tests are conducted in accordance with the requirements of the corresponding Test Specification, including the recording of results.
- System Tests are only performed once the prerequisite Tests have been completed and signed off.
- The completed System Tests are fully signed off by appropriate supplier (and possibly user) personnel.

### 5.5.4 User Compliance and Validation

It is the role of the user's Compliance and Validation (C &V) function to ensure that:

- The Test Strategy is appropriate to the GxP criticality of the system and the size and complexity of the system

- The need for the various System Test Specification(s) (and associated tests) are clearly defined in the Validation Plan or Test Strategy, along with the scope and outline content of the Specification (or the reasons for omitting or combining them).
- The need for and nature of reviewing and approving System Test Specification(s) and witnessing the System Tests by the user are clearly defined in the Validation Plan (the rationale for the review? Who reviews it? When do they review it? How do they review it? How they formally reject/accept? Who witnesses the tests? Who formally accepts the results of the tests?).
- The System Test Specification(s) are traceable to the Validation Master Plan, the Project Quality Plan, the Test Strategy and the corresponding System (Design) Specification.
- The level of user involvement in conducting/signing off the System Tests is clearly defined and justified in the Validation Plan.
- The acceptable level of System Test documentation is clearly defined in the Validation Plan or Test Strategy (details required, authorised signatories allowed to sign off the tests etc).
- The need to review the System Test documentation as part of the Qualifications (IQ, OQ and PQ) and the degree of the review is clearly defined in the Validation Plan or Test Strategy (including who reviews it, when and how they review it and how they formally accept or reject it).

### 5.5.5 Project Manager

It is the role of the user's and supplier's Project Managers to ensure that:

- All of the documentation required by the user's Validation Plan, the supplier's Project Quality Plan and the Test Strategy is developed in a timely and properly sequenced manner and to the required standard:
  - The System Test Specification(s)
  - The System Test Sheets(s)
  - The System Test Result(s)
  - Incident Reports (if required)
- All hold points are properly observed, and that user reviews are conducted before moving on to subsequent (dependant) phases of the project life cycle.
- The review of System Test Specification(s) is conducted prior to conducting the corresponding System Tests.
- The System Tests are conducted in a timely manner, all results are properly recorded and any necessary retests performed and signed off prior to moving onto subsequent tasks.
- Testing integrity is not compromised due to budgetary or time constraints.

### 5.5.6 Information Systems and Technology

It is the role of the supplier's Information Systems and Technology function to ensure that:

- The necessary test facilities and infrastructure are available to allow the System Tests to be conducted (i.e. network infrastructure, printers, test equipment, simulation software).
- The System Tests are properly supported as required (with regards to resources, facilities, witnesses etc.).

It is the role of the user's Information Systems and Technology function to ensure that:

- The necessary test facilities and infrastructure are available to allow the Site Acceptance Tests to be conducted (i.e. network infrastructure, printers, test equipment, simulation software).

### 5.5.7 Supplier Software Test Team

It is the role of the supplier's software testing function (the 'Test Team') to ensure that:

- The System Test Specification(s) are developed in a timely manner, and in accordance with the requirements of the user's Master Validation Plan and the supplier's Project Quality Plan.
- The System Test Specification(s) are submitted to internal review and approval as per the supplier's Project Quality Plan (and if required, by the user as per the user's Validation Plan).
- The System Test Specification(s) are traceable to the corresponding System (Design) Specification, the user's Validation Plan and the supplier's Project Quality Plan.
- Formal System Tests are conducted in a timely manner, in accordance with the corresponding System Test Specification(s).
- The results of all formal System Tests are recorded in accordance with the requirements of the corresponding System Test Specification(s).
- Any necessary retesting is conducted in a timely manner, in accordance with the requirements of the System Test Specification(s).
- All System Tests are signed off in accordance with the requirements of the System Test Specification(s).
- Incident reports are generated for any exceptional results or circumstances that are likely to have a wider knock-on effect and will need further consideration.

Note that it is good testing practice on large projects for one set of developers or engineers to develop the System (design) Specification(s), a different team to develop the System Test Specification(s) and possibly a third, independent team to conduct the actual tests.

This ensures that the System Testing is sufficiently thorough and that the expectations and preconceptions of software designers will not impact upon the conducting of the tests.

This is not always possible on smaller projects, but the preparation of good quality System Test Specification(s) will minimise any negative impact from using the same developers/engineers to both develop and test the functional design.

## 5.6 Relationships with Other Life Cycle Phases and Documents (Inputs and Outputs)

Figure 5.1 shows the relationship between the various validation and development life cycle phases and documents. Where appropriate the Test Strategy should clarify the project specific relationships. The various system Test Specifications are related to other documents in the life cycle and either use information from those documents as input (reference) data, or are in turn referred to by other documents and therefore provide output (result) data.

These related phases and documents are:

### 5.6.1 Validation Plan and Project Quality Plan

Where they include the Test Strategy, the Validation Plan or Project Quality Plan should explicitly indicate which specifications and corresponding Test Specifications should be produced (and tests conducted).

As a minimum, the Validation Plan should refer to the process of auditing the supplier to ensure that supplier tests are properly conducted and may also reference a supplier audit report that indicates the general nature and scope of these tests.

However, at the time of writing the Validation Plan for a large or complex system it is unlikely that the user will have sufficient idea of the system to be used to be able to define the tests in much detail (unless the user is implementing the system themselves).

The detailed requirements of the Test Specifications will more usually be deferred to the Project Quality Plan. In the case of large or complex projects a separate Test Strategy document may be produced, or the content may be included in the IQ, OQ and PQ Protocols.

Note that these interrelationships are summarised in a traceability matrix in Appendix G – Traceability Matrices.

### 5.6.2 Design Specification(s)

The various Design Specification(s) provide an increasing level of detail regarding the function and design of the system.

Design Specifications should be written in a structured manner, so that each separate function of the system is clearly described and can be individually tested. They should contain explicit, concrete details of functionality and design which can be tested and pass/fail criteria should be clearly identified — rather than implied).

As an example *The system will interface to a Schmidt Model 32X bar code scanner, capable of scanning and identifying 15 pallets per minute on a continuous basis* rather than *The system shall be capable of identifying a large number of pallets.*

When writing Design Specifications it is useful if:

- The corresponding Test Specification is written in parallel, almost certainly by a different person or team.
- A member of the test team reviews the Design Specification.

Both of these steps help ensure that functional and detailed design requirements are testable.

The relationship between a Design Specification, the corresponding Test Specification, and the Test Scripts should be identified as linked configuration items in whatever Configuration Management system is used. This ensures that if one document is changed the other(s) will be identified as part of any change control impact analysis and noted as requiring review and possible modification.

Note that these interrelationships are summarised in a traceability matrix in Appendix G – Traceability Matrices.

### 5.6.3 Tested Software and Hardware

Once tested at a low level (hardware and software module), the system hardware and software are a direct input to subsequent System Tests.

The tested software modules are outputs from the System Module Tests and inputs to the System Integration Testing.

The hardware is an output from the hardware testing and is an input to the System Acceptance Testing, along with the tested software.

Prior to conducting the System Acceptance Tests the system software should have successfully completed a thorough and challenging Software Integration Test. Likewise, the system hardware should have successfully completed Hardware Acceptance Testing. The

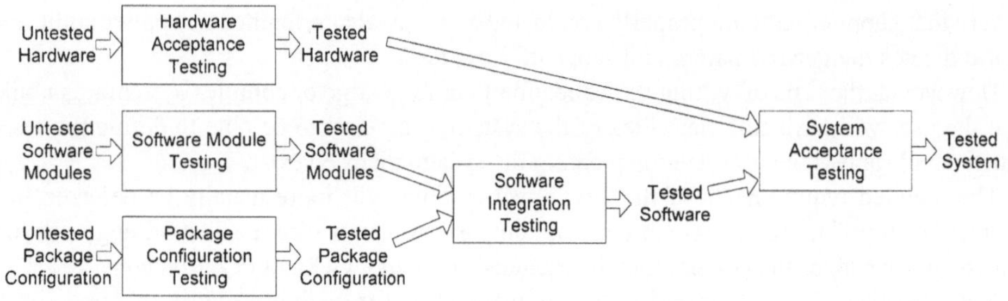


**Figure 5.3 – Output Tested Hardware and Software as Inputs to Subsequent Tests.**

purpose of the System Acceptance Test is to bring the actual system software and hardware together, and prove the overall functioning of the system in line with the requirements of the Functional Specification.

Since the previous Software Module and Software Integration Testing will have been conducted on the same (or functionally equivalent) hardware, the System Acceptance Testing should be a formal opportunity to demonstrate and document the overall functionality rather than conducting rigorous challenge tests (Figure 5.3).

It must be stressed that System Acceptance Tests should only be conducted once the underlying software and hardware have been tested and approved.

Note that these interrelationships are summarised in a traceability matrix in Appendix G — Traceability Matrices.

### 5.6.4 System Test Specification(s)

The System Test Specifications are used as inputs (reference documents) during the actual System Acceptance Testing.

They contain important information (as described below) and the System Test Specifications are therefore a mandatory document for conducting the System Tests. No tests can proceed until the relevant Test Specification document is reviewed and approved.

Note that these interrelationships are summarised in a traceability matrix in Appendix G – Traceability Matrices.

### 5.6.5 Factory/Site Acceptance Test Results and IQ, OQ and PQ

There is an increasing tendency to acknowledge that IQ, IQ and PQ Protocols and Reports (which have been adopted from process/equipment qualification) may not be best structured to report on a complex set of interrelated computer systems tests.

The focus should always be on documenting the rationale for the scope, nature and level of testing and on interpreting the test results. In this context Test Policies, Test Strategies and supplier FATs, SATs and User Acceptance Testing may serve a more useful purpose than more traditional IQ, OQ and PQs.

Installation Qualification protocols and reports are still a useful way of documenting the installed system and of bringing the system under Configuration Management. OQ and PQ are less useful and may be omitted if they serve no useful purpose (and if the validation policy allows this).

Where an organisation still requires a formal IQ, OQ and PQ to be conducted and reported upon, the emphasis should be on reducing the testing required solely to produce such documents. As described above, there may be a clear relationship between Factory and Site Acceptance Test results and the formal IQ, OQ and PQ Reports. Wherever possible, the IQ, OQ and PQ protocols should simply reference Test Strategies and Test Cases and IQ, OQ and PQ reports should reference the documented results of FATs and SATs.

Note that these interrelationships are summarised in a traceability matrix in Appendix G — Traceability Matrices.

CHAPTER 6

# The Development Life Cycle of a Test Specification

As with any formal process, there is a logical sequence to be followed when developing the System Test Specifications and when conducting the System Tests and there are recommended activities that should be included in order to assure successful completion of the testing phase.

These are described in the various sections in this chapter:

## 6.1 Recommended Phasing; Interfaces between and the Dependencies of Activities

It is recommended that the activities associated with developing the System Test Specifications and performing the System Tests be conducted in the order shown in Figure 6.1 in order to:

- Develop the System Test Specifications and conduct the System Tests in the most efficient manner.
- Provide sufficient traceability to ensure successful validation.

Certain of these activities have dependencies that require that they be carried out in a specific order. Where this is the case the two activities are shown in Figure 6.1 as being linked with a bold arrow and can be summarised as follows:

- The Validation Plan, Project Quality Plan and Test Strategy (Test Plan) must be completed before any other activity.
- The Functional or Design Specification must be completed before the associated Test Specification.
- The Test Specification must be completed before actual Tests take place.

This implies that any changes or updates to the prior activity must be reviewed to ensure that the impact upon all dependant activities is understood and any subsequent revisions carried out.

Many of the activities listed will have a formal or informal interface.

Formal interfaces may be required in the case of dependant activities, where one activity must be completed before a subsequent activity starts. This is usually the case when the sequence of the related activities is important in building a robust validation case.

In these cases the output from one activity is used as the input to the subsequent activity and this interface should be acknowledged and documented by referring to the prior activity in the documentation of the dependant activity.

It should also be remembered that some of these interfaces might be two-way. If problems are encountered in a subsequent activity it may be necessary to review some of the prior activities to see if any change is required. If this is the case any changes to the prior activity should always be reviewed for any impact upon ALL dependant activities, not just the one that initiated the change. Good Configuration Management will support this process. This is shown in Figure 6.1.

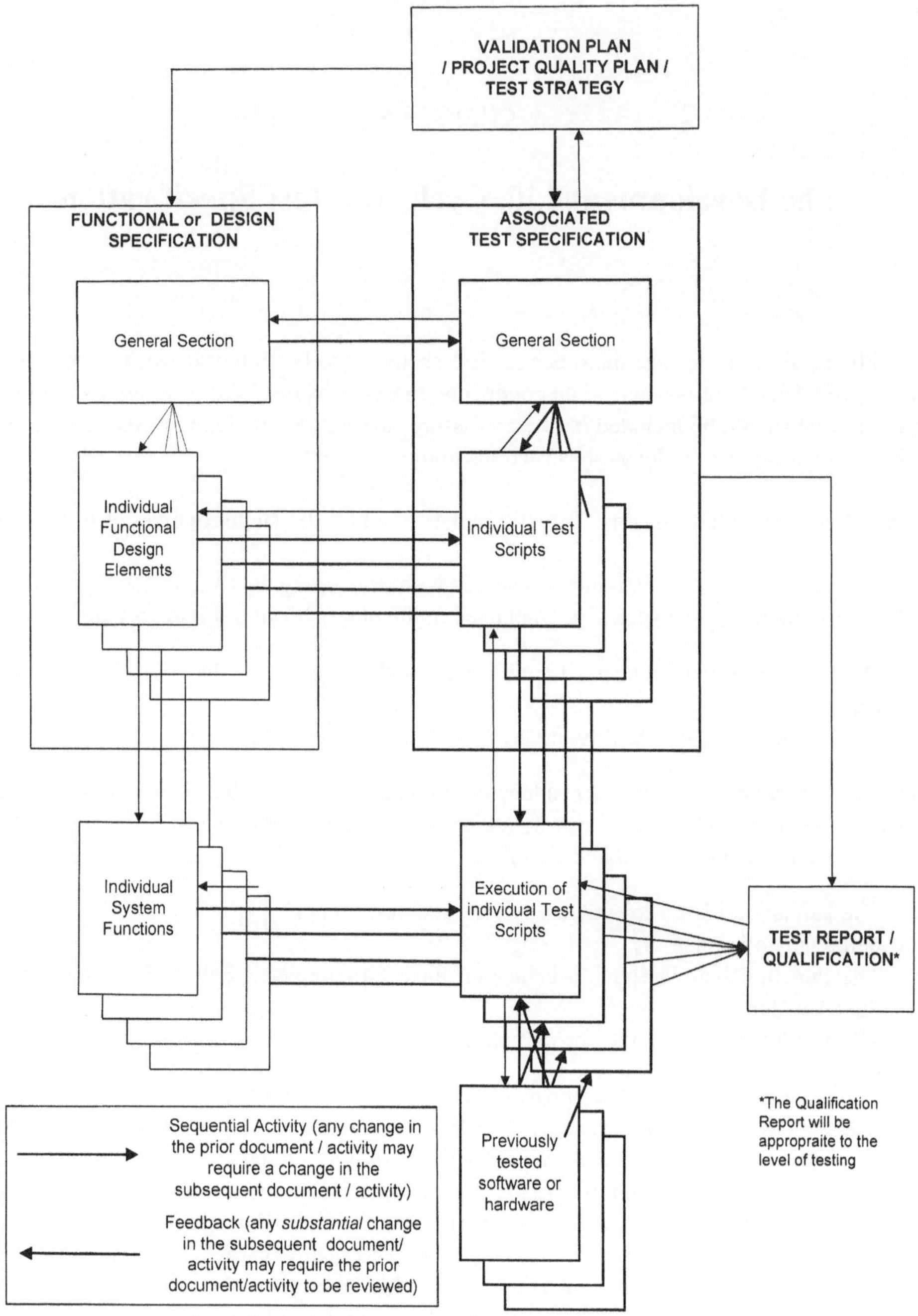


**Figure 6.1 – The Dependencies: Various Life Cycle Documents and Activities.**

## 6.2 Milestones in the Process

The major milestones in the development of a Test Specification and the conduct of the System Tests are:

- Completion of the first draft of the Functional or Design Specification (until which the development of the associated Test Specification can not start).
- Completion of the Functional or Design Specification (until which the associated Test Specification can not be completed).
- Development, review and approval of the individual Test Scripts (until which the associated System Tests can not start).

## 6.3 Inputs to the Development of a Test Specification

There are several inputs to the development of a Test Specification and checks should be made that all of the required input (reference) material is complete, approved and available before work on the related section of the Test Specification starts.

These inputs are listed in Section 5.2 but in summary come from:

- Validation Plan/Project Quality Plan
- Test Strategy
- Functional Specification

## 6.4 Document Evolution

The development of a Test Specification is an evolutionary process and, although sometimes overlooked by those responsible for their development, these documents are subject to review and approval.

This will be followed by the actual System Testing and the detailed sequence of this evolution is given in Figure 6.2. Note that although only two individual system tests are shown (1 to n), there may be any number of system functions under test at each stage of testing.

### 6.4.1 The Review Process

Each section of the document will be subject to review, as determined in the supplier's Project Quality Plan and possibly by the user's Validation Plan. Internal (supplier's) review may take the form of:

- Review by the author alone (not recommended)
- Review by peer(s)
- Open review, for instance, by a 'walkthrough' of the document by the author and peer(s)
- Review by a separate Quality Assurance function.

Depending upon the requirements of the Validation Plan, the user may be required to conduct a formal review of the System Acceptance Test Specification. This will be after the final internal reviews have been completed and may be limited to any, or all, of the following:

- Review of the general Test Specification only (to check general test principles and methodology).
- Review of a random number of individual Test Scripts (to check the quality of these).
- Review of all of the individual Test Scripts.

Note that it is unusual for the user to review and approve Test Specification and Test Scripts other that those for System Acceptance Testing.

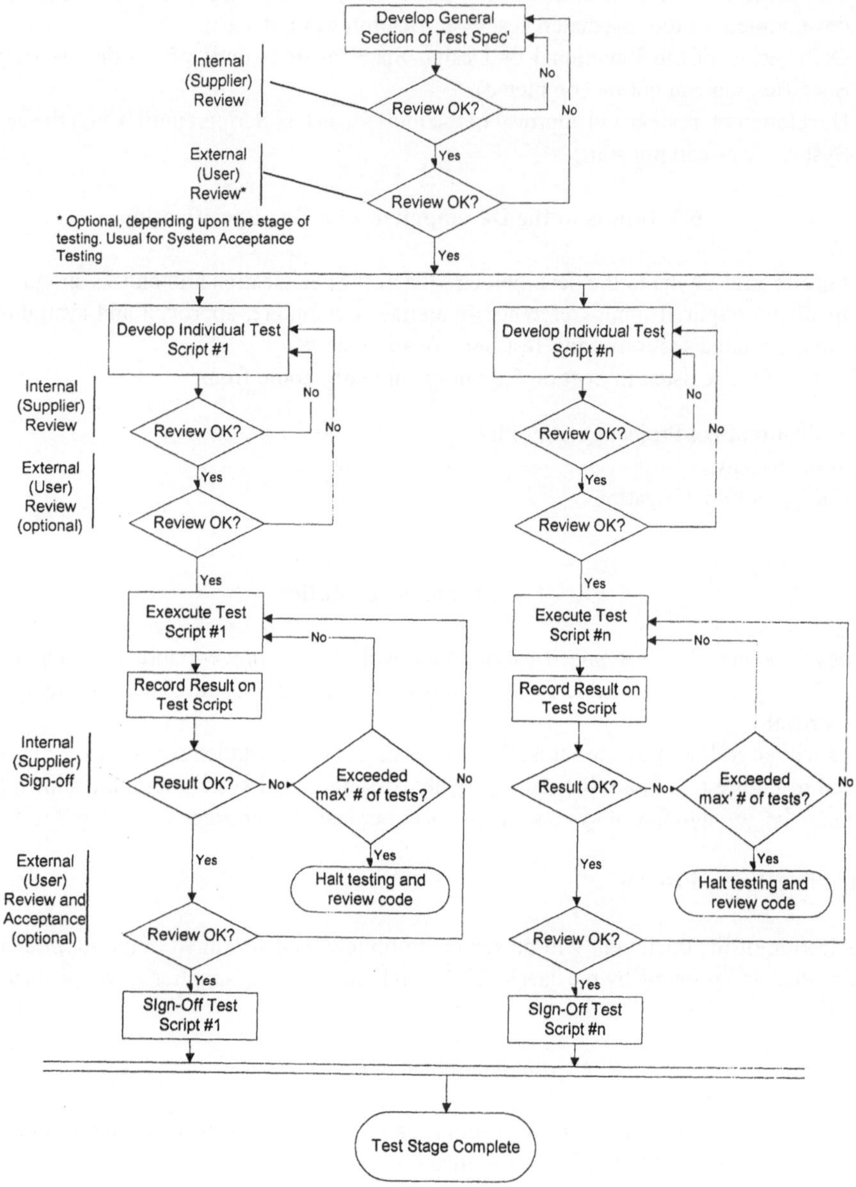


**Figure 6.2 – The Evolutionary Development of Test Specification and Associated Test Scripts.**

When conducting reviews the following points should be considered:

- Reviews should be conducted against the relevant input (reference) documents to check that the contents of the Test Specification meet the requirements for thorough testing of the system functions under test.
- Any assumptions that are not based upon the input documents should be challenged and either justified in the Test Specification or omitted.

- Where the Test Specification relies on information contained in the input (reference) documents full cross references are required (by page and paragraph or specific section number).

It may be necessary to conduct several iterations of the review process, possibly using more stringent review procedures for the final review. For instance, peer review could be used for initial and interim reviews, but open reviews could be used for the final review and approval.

Once the Test Specification has passed a review its status should be updated in the document register to reflect this.

## 6.5 Constraints on the Development of a Test Specification

There may be constraints on the development of a Test Specification and these are usually a lack of qualified personnel or the prerequisite input documents. This may either constrain the development of the entire document, or individual Test Scripts.

The effect of these constraints should be considered before commencing on any particular section of the document and unless the constraints can be overcome, work on the section must be placed on hold. Emphasis should always be on proper planning to ensure that the required resource and inputs are in place at the proper stage in the project.

Where a constraint is identified and a justifiable work-around is reached, it is suggested that the reasons for the initial constraint are documented in addition to the solution. This will provide the necessary level of traceability and it is suggested that the solution be discussed between the supplier and the user, so that the impact on the overall validation life cycle can be considered and the agreement of the user recorded in the project minutes.

## 6.6 Constraints on the Testing

There may also be several constraints on conducting the actual Software Integration Tests. These may either constrain all of the tests or just individual tests. These constraints can be anticipated, managed and overcome and some of these constraints (and solutions, if any) are defined in Table 6.1:

**Table 6.1 – Constraints on Testing**

| *Constraint* | *Solution* |
|---|---|
| The Test Script is not available (or finally approved). | Testing proceeds 'at risk', clearly stating any assumptions that are made in lieu of clear input (reference) material and with all test methods and results being fully documented. When the appropriate Test Script becomes available a full review of the Test must be held to determine whether or not the test and its results are valid. No test should be signed off until such a review is held. Note it is extremely unlikely that this will save any time! |
| Appropriate Test Equipment is not readily available. | Appropriate test equipment must be sourced from an alternative location, with full records being made of the test equipment used. |
| It is not possible to functionally test the system because of an inability to simulate input criteria at the supplier's factory. | Final System Acceptance Testing may be deferred until the system is installed on site (Site Acceptance Testing) |

## 6.7 Conducting the Tests

The individual functions of the system are part of the foundation of a quality installation, and properly conducted and documented System Tests are an integral part of successful validation.

Careful thought needs to be given as to how the tests can most efficiently be conducted and the methods, tools, equipment and personnel used. Further guidance on this is given below, throughout Section 6.7 as follows.

### 6.7.1 Test Methods

There are several different methods of conducting System Tests. Each 'method' will define a series of steps, conducted in a repeatable sequence in order to demonstrate that the functional objectives of the test(s) are met.

All of the individual tests may be conducted using the same methodology, or a variety of test methods may be used as appropriate to each test.

All tests consist of entering agreed test data as inputs to the system function and recording the resultant output data. This can be achieved in a variety of ways using a number of different test methods. If it is not possible to conduct such a predictable and repeatable test, the function will have to be verified instead of tested (see Section 3.4).

Each of the main test methods is described below, but it should be noted that this only provides an overview of these methods. The exact test methodology will still need to be described in the actual Test Specification, either in the General section, or in the individual Test Scripts.

The detail in which the test is described may vary according to the test methodology described in the General section of the Test Specification. It may be necessary to provide detailed step-by-step instructions (including providing full details of individual keystrokes for the test engineer to follow) or it may be acceptable to provide general instructions that rely on the test engineer using an overall knowledge of the system under test.

The basic principle to follow is that the level of detail included should allow the test to be repeated in exactly the same manner. For final System Acceptance tests it may be acceptable to allow the user (who should conduct the test) to follow the Standard Operating Procedure (SOP) to perform the actions required in the test. This has the added advantage that it tests not only the system, but also that the instructions in the SOP are aligned with the current version of the system and that the user's training is sufficient to allow the task at hand to be executed.

At many levels, the system functions under test are deemed to be unique and it is unlikely that any general training or documentation will refer to the function under test. This places specific emphasis on providing clear and unambiguous instructions, more so than for standard devices or manufacturing tests, which may rely on standard documentation and training for standard software and hardware modules.

Where full step-by-step details of the test method are not provided, the General section of the System Acceptance Test Specification should provide details of the necessary level of training required of the test engineer.

In this latter case it is acceptable for the individual Test Script to reference a General section of the Test Specifications. For example '*Select "box count" function, check that the control mode is in "Auto: and enter the number of boxes to count – refer to Section 2.1.1 of this specification: "Entering demand values" for specific instructions*'.

When defining the test methods to be used the following issues must be considered:

### 6.7.2 Manual Data Input

Data can be entered into the system function manually by a test engineer entering data into the system. The data to be entered will be specified in the individual Test Script and this will also describe how the information is to be entered (e.g. what order the data should be entered in, how long a 'wait' period should be employed, etc.).

*6.7.2.1 Manual recording of results*

Manual data input often requires the results of the test to be recorded manually, sometimes by observing a value on a screen or by observing an actual physical event (such as a pallet being delivered, or a new order being entered into a system). Since the purpose of the System Acceptance Testing is to check the actual functional performance of the system it is quite likely that system functions or actual physical actions will need to be observed and recorded.

In this case the individual Test Scripts should provide details of where and how the resulting data can be accessed or what is to be observed and should provide a place for the actual results to be recorded.

Note that results may be recorded qualitatively ('pass' or ' fail') or quantitatively (numerically, or any other quantifiable result such as a written word, error message, etc.). Where the test run will be subject to later review, results should be recorded quantitatively so that the independent reviewer can assess whether or not the test objective was met by achieving the recorded result.

Where the item or function under test has no direct impact upon product quality or data integrity, good testing practice may be followed and test results may be recorded in the form of a simple checklist (see Section 7.9).

*6.7.2.2 Physical simulation*

It may be acceptable or preferable for input data to be physically simulated. This might be appropriate where multiple values need to be changed 'simultaneously' and can be more easily achieved by the manipulation of physical devices (e.g. switches, potentiometers, etc.) connected via physical inputs to the system function under test. This may also be true where the functionality under test operates in the 'real world'. In these cases it may be necessary to physically simulate or operate a real piece of equipment or plant in a defined and repeatable manner (e.g. manually feed a pallet in an automatic palletiser or deliberately misfeed a label).

Where this is the case, detailed step-by-step instructions may also need to be given in the individual section of the Test Specification, or instructions in the General section of the System Acceptance Test Specification may be referenced as described above. For example '*Select bar code reader number 1 and scan the label on the tablet box – refer to Section 3.2.1 of this specification: "Using bar code scanners" for specific instructions*'.

As above, this method of testing usually requires the results of the test to be recorded manually, either by observing a value on a screen, by observing an output reading or status on an indicating device connected to the software function outputs or by observing an actual event. In this case the individual Test Scripts should provide details of where the resulting data can be accessed or observed and should provide a place for the actual results to be recorded.

*6.7.2.3 Software simulation/emulation ('Test Harness')*

For more complex system functions it may be acceptable or preferable to simulate or emulate the input data by using software. This may be the case where:

- The input data needs to be changed faster and with more accuracy than can be achieved manually.

- Where multiple inputs need to be changed in a precise pattern or sequence which cannot be achieved manually.
- Where it is not possible to enter values in any other way.

Simulation is usually used to refer to the process whereby multiple inputs to the system under test are calculated in real-time by a software model that simulates the process or function the system is controlling.

Emulation is usually used to refer to the process where the output from an external system (which is interfaced to the system under test) is replicated by a simpler system. Such emulation software can usually be controlled manually, allowing a wide range of interface conditions and data to be tested without relying upon setting up a large or complex external system.

The use of software 'test harnesses' is more usual when testing more complex system functions (as opposed to the simpler underlying software modules).

A well designed system will allow input and output parameters to be passed to and from the system function under test without requiring special 'test hooks' (this ability is 'inherited' from the underlying software modules and is often a function of a well designed system). In order to test the function a software test harness is developed to pass test parameters to and from the function under test (this is the software equivalent of a hardware test harness, which is traditionally connected to the system under test).

In this case the individual Test Scripts will reference the details of the test data (values, sequence, pattern) and the details of the simulation software and dataset(s) that will be used. This should include details of software version numbers.

Where a standard simulation routine is employed, its use can be described in the General section of the Test Specification and referenced by the individual Test Scripts. Where a specific piece of simulation software is used (which is more often the case for System Acceptance Testing) its development should be controlled and reviewed as part of the evolutionary process of developing the individual Test Specification.

The development of test datasets should also be controlled and reviewed in a similar manner and should be documented as part of the test results.

The recording of results from tests conducted using simulation software may either be done manually or automatically.

*6.7.2.4 Test datasets*

Where test datasets are used they are also subject to careful design and control.

The data included in such datasets should be carefully chosen to properly exercise the system function throughout its normal operating range. Where more that one set of input values is included in a test dataset the effect of the interaction between the input values needs to be carefully considered.

For example, it may be necessary to maintain one input at a constant value while changing another variable. A complete test dataset may include data which varies only one value at a time while maintaining all others constant and which may then move on to vary two or more values simultaneously.

A complete test dataset will exercise a system function at various points in its normal range. It is unusual to perform challenge testing as part of a System Acceptance Test, the purpose of which is to demonstrate the correct functioning of the system under test. Challenge (or stress) testing (outside of normal operating limits and ranges, using 'illegal' values) is more properly conducted as part of the Software Module or Software Integration Testing.

Test datasets should be included as part of the overall Test Specification review process and should be subject to change control when being developed and revised. Note that there are special considerations to bear in mind when the test data consists of data objects (this is covered in Section 7.17).

#### *6.7.2.5 Combined test methods*

Since the purpose of the System Integration and System Acceptance Testing is to test the functional performance of the system under test, it is often required to use a combination of test methods in a single test (manually input data, physically simulated data or data simulated by a software test harness). This allows a wider range of functionality to be tested, and may include physical simulation of parts of the plant or process, interfaces to external systems, etc. Where this is the case the appropriate test methodology should be clearly documented.

Specific attention should be paid to the sequencing of various input conditions generated by different methods of data entry. For example, attention should be paid to the timing of manually entered data when it is inserted amongst values generated by a test harness (software simulation). This will also be a consideration where test data is generated by different test harnesses that operate simultaneously.

#### *6.7.2.6 Automatic recording of results*

It may be advantageous to automate the recording of test results. This may be particularly appropriate where:

- There is a large amount of data to be recorded
- The output data needs to be recorded at a rate which is not possible by manual means
- There is a real possibility of errors being made recording complex data manually
- Results from an externally connected system need to be included in the test records

This is again more likely for Software Integration and System Acceptance Tests than for the simpler Software Module, Package Configuration or Hardware Acceptance Tests.

Wherever possible, the automatic recording of data should be accomplished using standard system facilities (data logging, alarm logging, trend data recording, etc.), which can be described in the General section of the Test Specification and referenced by the individual Test Scripts. This may also include the recording of outputs from the software function by a recording device attached to any physical outputs from the system.

If it is necessary to develop specific data recording applications these should be controlled and reviewed as part of the evolutionary process of developing the individual Test Specifications.

Some automatic recording systems or externally interfaced systems may not produce sufficient levels of documentation to provide traceability of the tests. For example, the time and date may not be included, nor the name of the variable(s) being recorded. Where this is the case additional documentation (usually in the form of manual notes) should be appended to the output (see Section 7.12).

Many computerised test management tools are able to automatically record results as part of their automated testing functionality.

#### *6.7.2.7 Automated testing*

Conducting the System Acceptance Tests can be a time consuming and expensive process given the need to fully test every system function. This task can be eased by the use of automated testing, performed by a computerised test management tool.

This basically combines the functions of software and process simulation and automatic data recording to fully automate the task of system function testing. Although such facilities lend themselves to the testing of many similar functions they can still be used to either conduct a single test at a time or can conduct many tests one after the other.

If it is necessary to develop specific automated testing applications these should be controlled and reviewed as part of the Test Specification(s).

*6.7.2.8 Control and validation of test methods and test harnesses*

It is important that appropriate test methods (sequence of actions) are selected in order to:

- Conduct the tests in the most efficient manner and thereby minimise project costs.
- Conduct tests of sufficient rigour to prove the proper functioning of the system under test and thereby ease the subsequent task of Operational and Performance Qualification and add value to the process of validation.

Most supplier organisations will have common test methods (sequences) for conducting similar tests to ensure that these objectives are met and these will often include defining the structure and order in which test harnesses will be used.

Wherever possible standard test harnesses (i.e. software functions for testing and recording) should be used, although this may not be possible for testing unique system functions. Where these test harnesses are standard features of the system under test (or of a dedicated external test system) and where these features of the system have previously been validated it will not usually be necessary to validate the methods used. Previous validation of such methods may, for example, have been on a similar project or by general use in the pharmaceutical industry.

Where special test harnesses have been developed, either for the project or for an individual system function, these methods must be validated in the same manner as the system under test.

It is important that a supplier has a Quality Assurance system that will record the development and status of such software test harnesses between projects. Such a system should record the development of the software, where the test harnesses have previously been used and validated, and any subsequent version changes. Without this system it is probable that project specific validation of the test harnesses will be required.

### 6.7.3 Formal Acceptance of Test Results

All tests must be formally accepted ('signed off') upon successful completion. Who signs these will be specified in the supplier's Project Quality Plan or the user's Validation Plan. There may be two levels of acceptance as follows:

*6.7.3.1 Signing off the system acceptance test (sign off by tester)*

It is essential that the person responsible for conducting the test should also sign off the actual test. This person must be a properly trained/experienced and qualified test engineer, and he/she must conduct the test from start to finish, as being responsible for following documented test procedure, and ensuring that actual test results are properly recorded, manually or automatically.

They should ensure that the recorded results comply with the acceptance criteria (details of acceptable and unacceptable test results should form part of the individual sections of the System Acceptance Test Specification).

By signing off the actual System Acceptance Test the responsible engineer is certifying that:

- The test was conducted in accordance with the documented test methods

- The test engineer conducted or supervised all parts of the test (supervising either another engineer or an automated test system)
- The test results were properly recorded and are accurate
- The test results were in compliance with the acceptable test results documented in the Test Scripts

When the test engineer signs off the test record, he/she must include his/her name and signature, and the date on which the test was conducted. It may also be necessary to record the test run number when a test has been repeated more than once.

Where the individual System Acceptance Tests are to be witnessed (either internally by the supplier's personnel or externally by the user's personnel) the witness should also sign (including his name, signature and date) to confirm:

- That they have witnessed or reviewed the results
- That the results are consistent with the documented acceptance criteria

More guidance on the requirements for signing executed Test Scripts is given in Sections 7.10 and 7.11.

*6.7.3.2 Approval of the tests*

As well as signing off the individual Test Scripts it may also be necessary to review and sign off the complete set of tests (or a subset).

This may be the case where:

- A specific stage of testing is complete (Hardware, Software Module, Package Configuration, System Integration or System Acceptance), or a subset thereof.
- The supplier wants to ensure that all of the Factory Acceptance Tests have been conducted properly before moving the system to site. This is to ensure that the site work and Installation Qualification are not started prematurely and that the Factory Acceptance Test documentation is of sufficient quality and consistency to facilitate the user's task of validation.
- The user wants to ensure that the test documentation is of sufficient quality and consistency to facilitate his own task of validation before proceeding to the next stage of testing.

This review may take several forms including:

- A review of some or all of the individual Test Scripts against the General section of the System Acceptance Test Specification. This is to ensure adequacy of cross referencing and consistency between tests.
- A review of some or all of the executed Test Scripts to ensure that the tests have been conducted properly, all results recorded properly, that the results were within expected ranges and that the tests have been properly signed off by the test engineer.

The review of the actual test procedure and results may be conducted in parallel with the conducting of the actual tests (the tester and the 'reviewer' sitting side by side). In this case the results sheets can be signed off by the reviewer just after the test engineer signs off the test records. More usually this can also take the form of a post-test review, where some or all of the test records and documentation is reviewed as a separate exercise (possibly by the users as part of the IQ).

Regardless of when the reviews of the test records and documentation are conducted, the reviewer should add their name, signature and date to the individual Test Scripts (usually when all tests are reviewed), or to a separate document which records which tests were reviewed (useful when a representative sample is reviewed).

## 6.8 Outputs from the Testing

The deliverables from a given phase of testing are:

- The approved Test Specification
- The executed Test Scripts, including results, raw data and any test evidence
- Incident reports documenting any deviations
- Change control records relating to any subsequent modifications, plus justifications and approvals

CHAPTER 7

# Recommended Content for System Test Specification(s)

The following sections describe the typical structure and content of a System Test Specification(s). This assumes that a given Test Specification consists of a General section and individual Test Cases.

In some instances (for large or complex systems) it may be preferable to develop Test Cases as separately reviewed and approved documents, which reference a common Test Specification. An example of this would be where many Software Module Test Scripts reference a single Software Module Test Specification. If this were the case the Software Module Test Specification would have to be approved prior to approving and executing individual Software Module Test Cases.

## 7.1 Overview

As the name suggests, the overview section of the document provides a brief summary of the document, including who wrote/developed the document, the review process by which the document is approved, the scope of the document and its relationship with other documents in the validation life cycle.

### 7.1.1 Front Page/Title Block

The ‘title block’ of the document should include the following information as a minimum:

- Project name
- Document title
- Revision number (subject to formal document release/control)
- Author(s)
- Approval signatures and context of approval (technical, quality/compliance etc)

### 7.1.2 QA Review Process

A section of the document will refer to the quality control/review/acceptance procedures which apply to the document. These procedures will usually refer to the user’s Validation Plan and/or the supplier’s Project Quality Plan and will not usually describe these procedures in detail.

### 7.1.3 Scope of Document

The scope and purpose of the document should be clearly defined, so that those with only a peripheral interest in the document can easily understand what the purpose of the document is, what it covers and what it does not. Where relevant this should refer to the Test Strategy.

This should include the following sections:

*7.1.3.1 Reference section*

The purpose of the Test Specification should be described, with appropriate reference to the other documents in the validation life cycle. This section may also refer to a general description of the life cycle given in the Validation Plan.

*7.1.3.2 Grouping and ordering of tests*

In a project with multiple system functions it is likely that tests will be ordered in a specific manner and may be grouped together. This implies that the tests themselves will be conducted in a particular order. The reasons for the particular ordering and grouping should be described, and may include:

- Conducting Factory Acceptance Tests before Installation Qualification and Site Acceptance Tests.
- Conducting simpler tests first and grouping similar tests together, thereby building familiarity with test methodology before moving on to more complex system functions.
- Test sequencing, where the output from one test is the input to the next test. This is important when the functional hierarchy means that more complex system functions are based upon simpler underlying system functions, which are in turn built using the base level software and hardware modules.
- Making most efficient use of common test resources (test equipment, personnel, etc.), prerequisites and set-up.

*7.1.3.3 Areas not tested and why*

It is possible that particular system functions, or some aspects of a particular function, may not be included in the System Tests (for instance, where a function or design feature is verified rather than tested – see Section 3.4). Where this is the case the reasons for not including a specific test in the series of System Tests should clearly be documented.

One reason for not testing individual hardware or software functions may be that the particular system function has previously been tested and validated on a previous project (either with the same or different users). Where this is the case the System Tests may be limited to:

- Providing full details of where and when the system function has been tested and validated before (referring to the users, Project, Test Specification and System Test records).
- Confirming that it is the same version of the system function and underlying software and hardware modules, running under the same operating system as previously tested/validated.

This is often the case with 'Commercial Off the Shelf' ('COTS') systems of known pedigree. Even where this is the case, details of any system functions not tested should be listed, along with the reasons for omitting the test.

*7.1.3.4 Bespoke test methods and harnesses*

Wherever possible, the testing of the system functions should follow a standard set of test methods that sequence standard test harnesses, or use standard methods for screen navigation, all of which are described in the System Test Specifications.

It is usual that the testing of many system functions will use different methods and harnesses, especially where the functional requirement or design feature tested is unique to the application or site. Where this is the case, the detailed methods and harnesses will be described in the individual Test Cases.

Possible reasons for using bespoke test methods and harnesses may include:

- It is impossible to test the system function using 'standard' test methods. This may be because the function under test is particularly complex.
- The testing of the system function combines several 'standard' test methods (for instance, where some inputs are simulated by software test harnesses, but where a few inputs are easier to simulate manually).
- Where actual physical simulation is needed, requiring part of the physical process or plant to be simulated or reproduced.
- Where interfaces to external systems are a large part of the functions under test.

## 7.2 General Section

In order to reduce the size and complexity of the individual sections of a System Test Specification (Test Cases) it is recommended that a General section of the System Test Specification be used to document common terms, principles, methods and prerequisites.

The following sections may be included in the General section of the System Test Specification and should be referred to by the individual sections of the System Test Specification (Test Cases) whenever relevant.

### 7.2.1 Glossary

The glossary should list and define all of the common terms that are used in the System Test Specifications and the test records. It is possible that this section refers to a common testing glossary, or one maintained as part of another project document, or to a standard glossary maintained by the supplier and user.

However, it is most likely that a project specific glossary will be used (or referenced) since it is likely that this will combine the agreed terminology of the user and supplier.

### 7.2.2 General Principles and Test Methodology

Because many of the System Tests will test similar system functions of similar complexity, these functions can be tested using a small set of principles using defined test methods and harnesses.

These common principles should be clearly described.

#### *7.2.2.1 Principle of testing*

The general test principles will document the overall nature and objectives of the tests and will describe how 'challenging' the tests will be. This will be specific to a given level of testing, or may describe how a standard test strategy (see Section 3.3) is applied to a particular system.

For instance, in the Software Module Test Specification this section may state that the principle is to conduct stress testing for all bespoke software modules with a high or medium GxP criticality (i.e. to try to 'break' the modules by using out of range data). It may also state that this will not be performed for bespoke software modules of low or no GxP criticality.

For the Software Integration Test Specification this section may state that the principle is to conduct stress testing for all software functions with a high or medium GxP criticality (i.e. to try to 'break' the modules by attempting to conduct illegal process in the work flow). It may also state that this will not be performed for software functions of low or no GxP criticality and that only normal process workflow will be demonstrated for these functions.

Where applicable, this may reference a relevant section of the Test Strategy.

*7.2.2.2 Standard test methods and harnesses*

The general description of the test methods to be used should be included in the General section of the System Test Specifications. This may include a general description of each of the test methods and test harnesses employed during the complete series of tests.

Including (or referring to) detailed instructions in the General section of the System Test Specification means that detailed instructions need not be given in every individual Test Case. This allows the individual Test Cases to focus on the functions under test and the expected (acceptable) results.

The individual Test Cases can, therefore, refer to the General section of the Test Specification and need not provide detailed instructions for every part of the test.

Descriptions should be provided for each type of test that will need to be conducted. As described, these may include methods for:

- Manual data input
- Physical simulation (including process or plant)
- Software simulation (including details of which software test harnesses to be used and how they will be used)
- Combined test methods
- Automated testing

As well as describing the different test methods this section should include references to:

- Any common documents such as operating manuals relating to the system under test. This should explicitly list references to the separate sections referring to operations such as:
  - Entering (simulating) analogue input values
  - Entering (simulating) digital input values
  - Enter (simulating or emulating) string (text) data
  - Changing set points
  - Changing the mode of control loops (auto, manual etc)
  - Etc.
- Any common documents providing instructions for:
  - Operating test equipment required to simulate physical inputs and display the status of physical outputs
  - Setting up and running software required to simulate inputs
  - Setting up and running automated test software
  - Operating process or plant required to conduct the System Acceptance Tests

If standard documents are not available for reference purposes then detailed instructions for conducting each type of test should be given. Although the General section only provides generic descriptions for each method of testing (which can then be referenced by simply including a 'tag number', point or channel number, function name, etc.), sufficient details should be included to allow any suitably qualified, trained or experienced engineer to conduct the test.

It is more usual to have to provide specific test descriptions and instructions for the type of Functional Testing included in the System Acceptance Tests. This is because the individual tests tend to be unique to the application and site. When it is required to describe the detailed test methodology to be used it may be necessary to include specific, step-by-step instructions including:

- The actions the test engineer has to take, such as:
  - Step-by-step keystrokes to be entered into the system under test
  - Step-by-step actions to be taken using physical input simulation equipment ('test rigs')
  - Step-by-step instructions describing the physical actions external to the system (to do with associated process or plant equipment)
  - Step-by-step keystrokes to be entered into the system simulating inputs or executing automated tests
- The acceptance criteria for the tests (see Section 7.2.2.3)
- How the results should be recorded (see Section 7.2.2.4)

The test methods and harnesses described in this section will be applicable to the majority of the individual tests at a given level of testing and all instructions should be clear, unambiguous and use language which is not subject to differing interpretations. Any ambiguity should be picked up as part of the review process.

*7.2.2.3 Acceptance criteria*

The basic purpose of testing is to ensure that the system functions in accordance with the applicable Design Specification. This means that the function under test will produce repeatable and predictable outputs for defined sets of input criteria.

The individual Test Scripts will clearly define the input criteria to be used in the test and these should produce a predictable set of output criteria. The predictable outputs are defined as 'acceptance criteria' and the purpose of the test is to ensure that the output of the system function matches the expected acceptance criteria.

In order for a test to serve a useful purpose, every test should have a defined set of unambiguous acceptance criteria for each set of defined input conditions. In the case of Functional Testing the acceptance criteria may be described (at least in part) in terms of the actual physical process, plant or equipment controlled or manipulated by the system under test. Examples include the emptying of a reactor, the stacking of pallets or even data being transferred between two external systems.

The way in which the acceptance criteria are defined and documented should be described in the General section of the System Test Specifications, and the actual acceptance criteria should be clearly documented for each individual test in the Test Script.

*7.2.2.4 Recording of results*

As well as providing a description of the test methods to be used it is important that details are provided of how results are to be recorded. This may include a description of the following recording methods:

- Manual recording of results
- Automatic recording of results.

Where results are recorded manually, a description should be provided which details:

- Where the data are recorded (usually on a standard test sheet, or possibly in a test database)
- To what accuracy data should be recorded (generally to the same accuracy as is given for the expected results).

Where data are recorded automatically information should be provided which details:

- The version of the recording software used (there may be more than one recording application used).
- The instruments to be used to record the status of physical outputs or external parameters (including the calibration details, model number, version number and connection details).
- Where the results will be stored (file name and format in the case of software records, or where a physical record may be stored when not attached to the test record).
- How the results will be 'passed' by the test engineer (by comparison to the defined acceptance criteria and by recording on a physical record sheet referring to the data, by an electronic signature attached to the data file, etc.).
- How the data can be 'played back' or recalled, including full operating instructions and details of the software application to be used (name, description, version number, etc.). This may be necessary in order to allow the tests to be reviewed or for the user to audit the tests.

*7.2.2.5 Test acceptance and 'sign off' (approval)*

The General section of the System Test Specification should also provide details of how the individual Tests Scripts should be signed off. This may require some or all of the following:

- Tests are 'signed off' by a nominated test engineer.
- Tests are reviewed at the same time the test is carried out ('witnessed') by a separate member of the supplier's test team
- Tests are reviewed at the same time the test is carried out ('witnessed') by a member of the user's project or validation team.
- Tests are subject to separate review by a member of the supplier's quality team.
- Tests are subject to separate review by a member of the user's validation team (possibly as part of the Operational Qualification).

### 7.2.3 General Test Prerequisites

Most tests will have some prerequisites that need to be in place before the test can be conducted. While some tests will have prerequisites that are specific and unique to the individual test, general prerequisites should be described in the General section of the System Acceptance Test Specification.

These may include

*7.2.3.1 Required system 'hardware' and software*

Details of the system hardware and software required to conduct the System Acceptance Tests should be given. For System Acceptance Tests, this should always be the hardware on which the Hardware Acceptance Tests were conducted. This may also be applicable to Software Module and Software Integration Tests that are hardware dependent.

The General section of the System Test Specification should list:

- Hardware that the tests should run on (usually just serial numbers at this stage). These should be checked against the versions recorded as part of the Hardware Acceptance Test.
- Software version numbers of all standard system software components (GAMP level 1 and 2 software) installed on the system that the tests should run on. Where applicable, in cases where 'hardware' is defined as including firmware and/or operating systems, this should be checked against the versions recorded as part of the Hardware Acceptance Test.
- Software version numbers of all system software modules (GAMP level 3, 4 and 5

software) installed on the system that the tests should run on. These should be checked against the versions recorded as part of the Software Integration Tests.
- Connection details of an appropriate test system configuration, including any data loggers, recorders, system printers, consoles, etc.

Where appropriate, references to specific operating instructions and the applicable level of experience, training or qualifications required to set up and use the equipment should be given.

*7.2.3.2 Required test equipment*

Details of the test equipment required to conduct the test should be listed. This will usually detail general equipment required to conduct a large number (or all) of the tests and may include:

- Equipment required to physically simulate inputs to the system under test (so called 'test-rigs').
- Equipment required to show the status of physical outputs from the system under test (so called 'test-rigs').
- Individual test instruments (meters, signal generators, oscilloscopes, logic probes, protocol emulators, etc.).
- Separate systems required to simulate software inputs to the system.

Where appropriate, details of the model and version numbers should be provided, along with references to specific operating instructions and the applicable level of experience, training or qualifications required to use the equipment.

Details should also be provided on how the equipment should be tested and how it should be set up for each specific type of test. Where reference cannot be made to specific operating instructions detailed instructions should be provided.

*7.2.3.3 Required test software*

Where tests are conducted using simulation software or automated test software, details of the software to be used should be given. This will include:

- Details of specific application software to be used, including application name, functional description, version numbers etc.
- Details of the hardware that this test software should execute on.
- Details of the individual Test Script, including unique name and version number.
- The change control procedures relating to the Test Scripts, including the author, version control and review procedures.

Where appropriate, references to specific operating instructions and the applicable level of experience, training or qualifications required to set up and use the software should be given.

*7.2.3.4 Required test datasets*

It is possible that multiple tests can be carried out using common sets of data. Where this is the case, the details of the test datasets should be provided in the General section of the System Test Specification.

These details may include:

- Which type of tests the individual datasets are applicable to

- The principle behind the test datasets (i.e. testing under and over range values, values across the valid range)
- The details of the test data (format, filename and location, number of values and possibly the actual values)
- The change control procedures relating to the datasets, including the author, version control and review procedures.

Because some or all of the software functions under test may be 'unique' it is sometimes useful to develop specific datasets for individual tests. Where this is the case all of the details above will apply.

*7.2.3.5 Required process, plant or equipment*

Because the System Acceptance Testing is a functional test of the system, it is sometimes necessary to test the operation of the system by reproducing part of the process, plant or equipment that the system is connected to.

Some types of process, plant or equipment can be simulated by software, using a scaled down or simplified physical model, or by an approximation of the 'real world' items being controlled or manipulated. Other items are more critical and lend themselves to actual testing in the supplier's factory. Examples may include a packaging line being fed with real product, labels, containers, etc. or an automated robot identifying, picking and transferring real product as part of the test.

Where process, plant or equipment are being reproduced or simulated, details of how this is achieved should be given. Where the test does not fully reproduce the functioning of the real site installation, this should also be described so that these shortcomings can be picked up during Site Acceptance Testing and/or Operational Qualification.

*7.2.3.6 Required test documentation*

Tests should always be conducted with the proper test documentation available and the standard prerequisite documents can be listed in this section. Common documents required to conduct the individual System Tests are:

- The approved System Test Specification
- A copy of the individual Test Script relating to the system function under test (part of the Test Specification, or as a separate document)
- Any related documentation referred to in either the General section of the System Test Specification or the individual Test Script (e.g. operating manuals)
- Test Record sheets to allow the results of the test to be recorded, reviewed and 'signed off' (if separate from the Test Script)
- Incident Reports, for any prior deviations which may impact in the test

*7.2.3.7 Test sequencing*

Although different system functions should be independent of each other, it may be desirable to conduct some tests in a preferred order in order to maintain testing efficiency.

Where general prerequisites exist for conducting prior tests these may be documented in the General section of the System Test Specification (see Section 5.6.3).

### 7.2.4 Appendices

Finally, the System Test Specification may contain any necessary appendices.

These will usually be information that does not bear directly upon specifying or conducting the general or individual tests, but will be useful background or reference material.

Example of information contained in an Appendix could be:

- A standard Units of Measure table for the system under test
- A bibliography of useful reference documents (such as various GAMP documents and guidelines)
- A full listing of the other related life cycle documents, including title, the latest version number and status
- A reference to the supplier's relevant Quality Assurance standards
- Etc.

## 7.3 Individual Test Cases

As well as a General section, the System Acceptance Test Specification will also contain details for all the individual System Tests that need to be carried out. These are often referred to as Test Cases.

The Test Cases will provide additional information, building on the General section of the Test Specification to give the final details on the purpose of the individual test, the functions that are to be tested, the expected results, etc.

The level of detail included in the Test Case should be relevant to the GxP criticality of the item under test. For items with no direct impact upon product quality or data integrity the Test Scripts may follow general industry good testing practice.

The following sections document the level of detail generally required for testing items, which has a direct impact on product quality or data integrity in systems of high or medium GxP criticality. In all cases the level of detail included in the Test Script should be appropriate to the GxP criticality. For each item of hardware, software, or system function the following items may be included in the corresponding Test Case:

### 7.3.1 Unique Test Reference

Each test should be given a unique reference, which identifies it as a separate entity. This may be the name of the system function under test (i.e. Centrifuge Operation) or may be some sort of code (i.e. CFG001).

This unique reference should be used whenever reference is made to the test in order to avoid any possible ambiguity.

### 7.3.2 Name of Hardware Item, Software Module or Function under Test

For Hardware Tests or Software Module Tests, the item of hardware or software module under test should always be clearly identified.

For Package Configuration, Software Integration or System Acceptance Tests, if the system function under test has a unique reference that does not explicitly identify the system function under test (i.e. CFG001) the name of the system function should always be included as an additional point of reference (i.e. Test CFG001 – Centrifuge Operation). Note that to avoid ambiguity the name of the function under test should always refer to the function as defined and referenced in the appropriate Design Specification.

### 7.3.3 Cross Reference to Functional Description or Design Detail

The functional description or design detail under test should always be identified as an individual section of the relevant Design Specification. This section should be explicitly referred to in the Test Script, including document name, revision number, section and possibly page and paragraph number.

It may also be desirable to include excerpts from the individual section of the Functional Specification if this eases the task of explaining the functions that are under test although this requires particular attention to be paid to change control procedures to ensure that the excerpt is maintained and up-to-date.

### 7.3.4 Specific Prerequisites

It is possible or even likely that some or all of the individual Test Scripts will have specific prerequisites that are not covered under the General section of the Test Specification. As described above, these may be categorised as follows:

- System Hardware and Software
- Test Equipment
- Test Software
- Test Datasets
- Required Process, Plant or Equipment
- Test Documentation
- Prior Tests

For the sake of efficiency, test prerequisites should be included in the General section of the System Test Specification wherever possible. The prerequisite section of the individual Test Script should only include:

- Specific details which 'instance' the general prerequisites (for example, a reference to the General section on test dataset prerequisites and then the name of a particular test dataset file from a common directory).
- Specific details which are unique to the individual test (for example, the use of a particular piece of equipment that is used for a single test).

### 7.3.5 Particular Test Methods and Test Harnesses

Specific details of the actual test methods and test harnesses used for the individual test must be given. This should include the following.

*7.3.5.1 Test objectives*
A brief description of the test methods should be given, for example:

- 'This test will check that the module rejects out-of-range input data, alerts the operator by providing a error message and logs the error'.
- 'This test will check the capability of the system to recognise when product boxes are incorrectly loaded into the feed mechanism' or
- 'This test will examine the correct functioning of Centrifuge Emergency Stop routines'.

*7.3.5.2 Methods used*

A detailed method (sequence) for conducting the individual test should be given, either by:

- 'Instancing' a test method described in the General section of the System Test Specification (for example, 'By using the test methods described in Section 2.3.7 — 'Entering Manual Instructions', instruct the robot to transfer 6 pallets from the inflow stack to the return stack'.)
- Describing in detail the methods used to conduct a unique test.

*7.3.5.3 Test harness used*

Details of the software test harness used to simulate inputs and 'read' outputs should be given, including the revision number of the test harness. This may either:

- Refer to a standard test harness (for example '*Use the Batch Record Data Test Harness to simulate finished product values and confirm that the system should create a completed batch record – see Section 3.1[a] for details of using the batch record system*'.)
- Describe in detail the use of a specific test harness developed for an individual test.

*7.3.5.4 Detailed instructions*

Where detailed instructions for conducting a unique test need to be provided, these should provide complete, step-by-step instructions in order to ensure repeatability in the way the test is performed. This will often be necessary to avoid ambiguity in the case of unique functional tests.

These are as detailed above for the general methodology section and, as a reminder, may include:

- The Principle of Testing
- The method(s) of testing employed:
  - Manual data input
  - Physical simulation
  - Software simulation (the use of a unique test harness)
  - Combined test methods
  - Automated testing
- Detailed reference to applicable documentation
- Step-by-step actions taken by the test engineer
- Equipment to be used
- What feedback or results to expect
- How the results should be recorded

### 7.3.6 Acceptance Criteria

For each test, details need to be provided on what constitutes a 'pass' and what constitutes a 'fail'.

This is done by providing a list or description of expected (acceptable) results. It is most useful to define only the acceptance criteria and to define any other result as a failure.

However, there may be occasions where there is a wide range of acceptable results, and a relatively small number of unacceptable results. On these occasions it is sometimes useful to provide a smaller list or description of unacceptable results so that a 'failure' can clearly be identified.

There should be no ambiguity between what constitutes a 'pass' or a 'fail' and there should be no 'middle ground' between the two.

This places the emphasis on identifying concrete, observable parameters than can be observed by the test engineer and upon using precise language to describe them. The appropriate Design Specification should be the basis for defined acceptance criteria. This should describe the User Functional Requirements or Design Details clearly enough to allow acceptance criteria to be identified.

Acceptance criteria should be clearly and unambiguously defined. For Software Module, Hardware and some System Integration Testing this can often be done by providing a specific acceptable value or list of acceptable values. In the case of a list of acceptable values, it is useful to document the acceptance criteria against the applicable input parameters in the form of a table.

Some System Integration, Package Configuration and all System Acceptance Tests are functional tests and the acceptance criteria may be given by providing a description of the expected results.

Note that the location where the results will be displayed should be described as part of the test methodology (which may be a physical observation) and that the acceptance criteria is usually a simple value, result list or description under a suitable header.

It may also be that the definition of acceptable performance may be clearly described in the Functional Specification. In this case a written description of function may form part of the acceptance criteria.

Examples of various acceptance criteria are given below:

- 'List of Expected Results – Hardware Test'

| *Input Values (mA)* | *Acceptable Results (mA)* |
|---|---|
| 0 | 4 |
| 4 | 4 |
| 12 | 8 |
| 20 | 20 |
| 24 | 20 |

- 'List of Expected Results – Acceptance Test'

| *Input Values*<br>*# Input Pallets* | *# Output stack pallets* | *Acceptable Results*<br>*# Pallets transferred* |
|---|---|---|
| 1 | 0 | 1 |
| 2 | 8 | 0 |
| 4 | 4 | 4 |
| 6 | 4 | 4 |
| 8 | 0 | 8 |

- 'The system will automatically increase the centrifuge speed from rest to a minimum speed of 3,000 rpm over a period of between 1 minute 30 seconds and 2 minutes. The centrifuge will run at a minimum speed of 3,000 rpm for a period not less than two minutes and not exceeding 2 minutes fifteen seconds. The centrifuge shall then decelerate, reaching rest in not more than 30 seconds.'

| | |
|---|---|
| Acceleration Time (> 1m: 30s, < 2m: 00s) | |
| Speed achieved | |
| Run Time (> 2m: 00s, < 2m: 15s) | |
| Minimum speed sustained | |
| Deceleration time (< 30s) | |

### 7.3.7 Data Recording

As well as defining the test methodology and the acceptance/failure criteria, it may also be necessary to detail how the results of the individual test should be recorded. This is usually the case where results are not simply written on (or entered into) a copy of the Test Script.

As with other sections, the details of how the data is recorded for the individual tests can either be by:

- 'Instancing' a recording method described in the General section of the System Test Specification (for example, 'by manually recording the test results as described in Section 4.3.4 – 'Recording the results of a compared floating point values', the results of the test will be recorded on the unique test sheet, signed and witnessed').
- Describing in detail the recording methods used to record the results of a unique test.

Where it is required to describe in detail the recording method to be used for a unique test, full details of how the information is to be recorded should be given (as described above in the paragraphs relating to the general data recording section).

### 7.3.8 Further Actions

It is possible that additional actions may be performed once the actual test is completed and signed off. Although not all of these are absolutely necessary from a validation point of view, additional information may be included in the individual Test Script. For instance, it may be necessary to make a piece of equipment or process plant safe following the execution of a test.

*7.3.8.1 Repeating failed tests*

It may be useful to describe how a test would be repeated if it does not pass the first time. This is useful in cases where it is not necessary to repeat all of the set up steps if the test is repeated immediately. It should be emphasised however that the purpose of the System Acceptance Test is to demonstrate the correct functioning of the system, and failed tests should be rare at this stage in the project life cycle.

It may also be useful to place a maximum on the number of 'repeats' that can be performed before a system function is deemed to have failed the test. For instance, it may be acceptable to repeat a test if the cause of the failure was a simple set-up error by the test engineer (a software module was left in manual when a complex control loop was tested, for example).

However, there is little benefit in repeating the same test numerous times if the problem is not immediately obvious, and it is useful to limit the number of tests that may be performed before a review of the underlying software and hardware test status and code is carried out.

It will also be necessary to specify that details on the cause of the failure must be recorded and where and how they should be recorded ('incident reports'). These can again 'instance' the General section of the System Acceptance Test Specification or provide unique, step-by-step details.

*7.3.8.2 Reset actions*

It may be necessary to perform certain reset actions to return the system to normal conditions following the execution of certain tests.

These reset actions can be defined in one of two ways:

- As a check to make before the individual test is conducted (to check the prerequisite status of the system/software).
- As a series of reset steps or actions to be conducted after each test.

Either of these methods may again either 'instance' the General section of the System Test Specification or provide unique, step-by-step details of the tests or actions to be performed.

*7.3.8.3 Preparation for next test(s)*

It may be desirable to detail any actions that could usefully be carried out to prepare the system/software for any following tests. This is, however, unusual since it is more flexible to include any specific set up instructions as part each individual test.

If this is the case, it is again possible to either 'instance' the General section of the System Acceptance Test Specification or provide unique, step-by-step details of the actions to be performed.

### 7.3.9 The Use of Separate Test Record Sheets

In many instances, a complete copy of the Test Script will be used to record the results of an executed test. However, there may be instances where the test may be complex and the specific instructions, prerequisites, etc. take many pages. In this instance it may be useful to have a separate Test Record Sheet. This makes the paper easier to handle during testing. The Test Record Sheet should have a 'header' page or section to document the test run number, the start time and date and the name of the tester. There should also be a footer section with space to indicate the completion time and date, a clear indication of the pass/fail status of the test and space to sign the test.

The main section of a Test Record Sheet usually is comprised of a table containing:

- The Test Step number
- The specific instruction to carry out (including details of any test evidence required to be taken)
- The expected result
- A space to write the actual result
- A space to write any comments or references about attached evidence, test incident sheets, etc.
- A space to initial the test step (including a witness if required)

The Test Record Sheets can either be sets of pages, bound in the main System Acceptance Test Specification, or may be separate sets of pages, usually kept in a loose leaf binder. The advantage of this is that the sheets for each test may be removed for ease of use and returned once the test is complete.

Where separate Test Record Sheets are provided, these should clearly reference the main Test Script and should be subject to full change control. Each page should contain details of the test (by unique test reference and name) as well as page numbers in the form of 'page N of M'. This is important since the individual Test Record Sheets may become physically separated from the main System Acceptance Test Specification and will need to be returned under proper control.

CHAPTER 8

# Good Testing Practices

Having established why we test, and what we should include in our tests (the Test Strategy), it is important to understand how to test, and what constitutes good testing practice in the healthcare industries. In previous sections we looked at some of the principles of testing and some of the techniques that can be used. There is, however, a human element to testing that also needs to be considered.

## 8.1 Prepare for Success

A successful testing programme begins well before testing commences. In many cases the testing is expected to make up for deficiencies elsewhere in the development programme; as the saying goes 'you can't test quality into a product'. Thought needs to be given to the testing programme from the moment the project starts, otherwise problems may well occur during the test execution.

## 8.2 Common Problems

It is possible to identify some common problems, to examine their causes and to consider what can be done to prevent them.

### 8.2.1 Untestable Requirements

In many cases the testing 'fails' because the User Requirements, Functional or Design Specification details were ambiguous, or were simply not testable. The obvious example is a User Requirements statement such as 'The system should be user friendly'. How is it possible to objectively test such a 'requirement'?

Requirements should be:

- Unambiguous – it should be clear what the requirement is and it should not be liable to differing interpretation.
- Testable – from reading the requirement it should be clear what can be tested to prove that the requirement has been met and what the test objective should be.
- Single stated – each requirement statement should contain only one requirement. In this way requirements can be proven in single Test Scripts, or in separate sections of a Test Script. Consequently, if a single requirement is not met during testing, the retest can be limited to that single statement. If long, complex requirements statements are produced (which is often the case from some techniques used to ascertain user requirements, such as question and answer sessions) and all of these are tested in a single long Test Script, the failure of any single point will require the complete test to be rerun.

- Itemised – each requirement should have a unique reference number or section number that can be referenced by the Test Script and cross referenced to the Test Script in a Requirements Traceability Matrix (RTM).

It is a failing with many 'accelerated' development methodologies ('Rapid Development Approach') that User Requirements do not meet these criteria because they are not sufficiently well documented. Even when 'accelerated' methods are used to capture User Requirements (question and answer sessions, conference room pilots, etc.) these should still be documented.

It is also very valuable to have an experienced tester review User and Functional Requirements, to ensure that they are sufficiently 'testable'.

### 8.2.2 Start Early

The writing of Test Specifications should be started early. As soon as a first draft of the relevant User, Functional or Design Specification is available, work should commence on developing the Test Strategy and the associated Test Specifications. This effectively means that the test team works in parallel with the development team.

Unless this is done, it is very likely that the test team will not be ready for testing once the development team has completed the building of the system.

This approach allows the structure of the Test Specification to follow the structure of the Functional or Design Specification, thereby introducing structure and logic into the testing programme. Note that the interrelationship between the test documents and the design documents should be included in the Configuration Management of the system, so that any changes in the Functional or Design Specifications will trigger a review of the relevant Test Specifications.

### 8.2.3 Plan for Complete Test Coverage

In many instances, the test team prepares a Test Programme to cover the items they feel are important, with little or no regard to the items that actually need testing. When designing the Test Programme, complete coverage of the User and Functional Requirements, and the Design Details should drive:

- What needs to be tested
- What the test objectives should be
- What Test Cases will cover each of the test objectives
- How the Test Cases will be organised and scheduled

Unless this approach is taken it is likely that requirements or details will be left untested, and that this will only be realised once testing is almost complete. This often leads to additional Test Scripts being developed at the last minute, which should be avoided if at all possible.

In accelerated development methodologies the standard test coverage usually only covers Functional Testing (System Acceptance Testing and some System Integration Testing at best). In these cases additional Test Scripts must be developed to conduct stress testing, challenge testing, user profile testing and so on.

Basically, Test coverage must meet the needs of the defined Test Strategy.

### 8.2.4 Insufficient Detail in the Test Scripts

Many accelerated development methodologies have standard 'off-the-shelf' test scripts but many of these have been designed for generic use across all industries. They are often unsuitable for use in the healthcare industries because they have:

- No place to record the reference to the requirement or detail being tested
- No place to record the test objective
- Insufficiently detailed instructions to set up the test
- Insufficiently detailed instructions to execute the test
- Ambiguous expected results, or no expected results at all
- No place to record results or the Test Script requires just a qualitative indication of test status rather than a quantitative record of the result
- No place to sign for each step or even for the complete test
- Insufficient room to record comments or references to attached evidence

These issues are covered in further detail later in the text, but the important issue is that a Test Script template must be produced which is suitable for supporting testing in a regulated Life Sciences environment.

### 8.2.5 Design Qualification – Start When You Are Ready

Testing is often seen as the 'catch-all' at the end of the development process, which will identify and resolve all sorts of errors in the software or system. Although one of the main objectives of testing is to do just that, this doesn't mean that the software or system should enter testing before there is a high degree of confidence in the quality of the software.

This can be achieved by following good development practices and by conducting a formal Design Review or Design Qualification, usually prior to the build commencing, but certainly before testing starts.

The criteria for releasing the design for testing should be established prior to the Design Review or Design Qualification commencing. The criteria can be included in a Design Qualification Protocol. Establishing the criteria prior to starting the review means that a baseline for acceptable design quality is established. It should be agreed that unless the acceptance criteria for the Design Qualification are met, testing would not commence. This is important since a risk-based Test Strategy will make certain assumptions on the development process and the quality of the design and testing will only be appropriate if these assumptions are met.

The Design Qualification may include requirements that:

- All items are under established Configuration Management
- Change Control is established for all Configuration Items
- Source Code Reviews have been conducted for all GAMP software category 5 code
- All source code is fully commented, including change history
- All Requirements and Specifications are up-to-date and approved
- The Requirements Traceability Matrix is fully populated and up-to-date

Where the development of the Test Programme has proceeded in parallel with the design, the Design Qualification may also include a review of the Test Specifications, Test Scripts, the traceability between Test Scripts and Requirements and test coverage traceability in the review. While this is certainly not a mandatory part of Design Qualification, it does increase confidence prior to testing.This ensures that testing is started with a high degree of confidence in the quality of the design and that the nature of the testing is appropriate to the design.

### 8.2.6 Taking a Configuration Baseline

If the worst happens, and the testing goes badly wrong, code gets corrupted or changed outside of change control, you will have to start some, or all, of your testing again.

In some organisations, although code, documents and so on will be formally approved at version 1.00 prior to testing starting, no formal baseline of the system configuration is taken until after the testing is complete. It is much easier to recover any documentation or code if the first formal baseline of the Configuration is taken prior to testing commencing. If there is a problem it is relatively easy to restore the baseline configuration and start again.

It is also good practice to take another baseline after each phase of testing. This means that the 'Configuration' of the system can be saved at a known point in time, limiting the amount of retesting needed if something does go wrong.

## 8.3 Testing in the Life Science Industries is Different

Many good Test Programmes, with an appropriate Test Strategy and well-written Test Cases, have been ruined because of poor testing practices. When a large number of human errors creep into a testing programme they call into question the outcome of individual tests and place the whole Test Programme into doubt. At best, certain tests will have to be repeated again, at worst the whole Test Programme may have to be repeated and in some cases projects have been cancelled because of poor testing practices.

This section looks at the human aspects of testing, and what can be done to maximise the chances of conducting a successful Test Programme in accordance with good testing practice.

One of the main problems when testing a large or complex system is that the size and complexity of the Test Programme often requires additional testers to be used. In many large healthcare companies there may be a core of people experienced in testing software based systems that are GxP critical.

This is not always the case in smaller companies or with suppliers who supply many different industries. Even in large healthcare companies contract resource may be used during the testing phase.

Testing in the Healthcare Industries is different from many others. There are four basic reasons for this:

- The testing may be more thorough than in other industries. This is because of the need to conduct 'challenge' tests to prove the integrity of the application.
- The content of the Test Scripts may be greater than in other industries (i.e. expected results must be clearly included on the Test Script, the Test Objective must clearly be stated, etc.).
- The level of proof required to document the test results may be higher than in many other industries (i.e. quantitative results must be recorded as opposed to a simple 'pass' or a tick in a box, witness signatures may be required).
- There is a need to assess the impact of any test failure or test anomaly with regards to the GxP impact or any changes required and the extent of any regression testing.

If people conducting tests are not used to working in this environment it is likely that they will make omissions or errors that will call the outcome of a given test into doubt. When this happens on a large number of test cases, it calls the validity of the complete testing programme into doubt.

Steps must, therefore, be taken to prevent this from happening.

## 8.4 Prerequisite Training

Unless the Test Programme is very short, or the entire team is familiar with testing GxP critical systems, it is worth investing time in providing some training before the Test Programme commences.

On projects that have slipped behind schedule there is often a tendency to rush into testing in order to 'make up for lost time'. This is, however, a false economy and the temptation should be avoided.

There are many advantages to providing such training, including:

- Training provides a useful breathing space for the team and allows them to ask any questions they have about the testing programme.
- It provides a basic introduction for those who have not tested in a GxP environment before.
- It also provides a useful refresher for those who have tested in the GxP environment before and who need to get into the right state of mind.

The training should cover:

- For those who have not tested in a GxP environment before, a session on 'regulatory awareness' (i.e. why systems are validated and why testing in the Healthcare Industries is different)
- An overview of the Test Programme
- Specific roles and responsibilities for those involved with the Test Programme
- Checking out and checking in of Test Scripts
- Conducting tests (executing Test Scripts)
- What to do in the case of a test error (i.e. something clearly goes wrong)
- What to do in the case of the test anomaly (i.e. something happens and you are not sure whether it is an error or not)
- The life cycle of a Test Script, from checking out, through execution, signing off, checking in and subsequent review.
- The life cycle of a 'test incident', including raising the incident, assessing the incident, closing the incident and retesting

It may be useful for these last two items to be demonstrated by stepping through the process using a real Test Script (although it is unlikely that this will constitute a real test execution).

A number of these topics are covered in outline in the following pages.

## 8.5 An Overview of the Test Programme

It is useful for the entire team to know what the overall Test Programme looks like. Everyone should understand the timing and especially the interdependencies that exist between different phases of testing and individual tests.

It should be made clear that although there will be target dates, the validity of testing must not be compromised in order to meet such dates. If tests are poorly conducted it is likely that they will have to be conducted again, thereby negating the benefit of 'meeting' target dates.

## 8.6 Roles and Responsibilities

There are a number of roles that various people will play in a Test Programme. Everyone on the team should know what the roles are and who is fulfilling each of those roles. These are described briefly below. The 'title' and scope of each role may vary between organisations, from Test Programme to Test Programme and, in small Test Programmes, one person may fulfil multiple roles.

### 8.6.1 Test Manager

The Test Manager is responsible for managing the overall Test Programme. This includes:

- Assigning the execution of Test Cases to Testers (and witnesses)
- Monitoring the progress of testing against the programme
- Ensuring test errors and anomalies are resolved at an adequate rate.

Further detail on this role is given in Section 8.7.

### 8.6.2 Lead Tester

On a large Test Programme there may be a Lead Tester who supports the Test Manager from a technical perspective. This person is usually an experienced tester, familiar with the process of testing in a GxP environment. If other testers have queries on the process of testing they should seek advice from the Lead Tester in the first instance.

The Lead Tester needs to maintain an overview on technical issues associated with the testing process, such as maintenance of test datasets in the correct status (see Section 8.17), the correct sequencing and execution of tests and the appropriate use of techniques and any tools that are used to support the testing process.

### 8.6.3 Tester

As the name implies, a Tester is responsible for the execution of individual Test Scripts, including the recording of the test results and capturing sufficient evidence. They should have experience of testing in a GxP environment or should have been adequately trained.

### 8.6.4 Test Witness (or Reviewer)

Some tests will require the use of a Test Witness; typically where insufficient proof can be captured. The witness may be a tester who witnesses other tests. Alternatively, key tests such as System Acceptance Tests may be witnessed by the user or client. See Section 8.11 for further information.

### 8.6.5 Quality/Compliance and Validation Representative

It is important that resources are available from either the supplier's Quality organisation, the user's Quality organisation or the user's Compliance and Validation organisation. The specific role that each will play will be determined on a project-by-project basis, by the contractual relationship. This should be defined in the Validation Plan or the Test Strategy. Their availability and involvement at the time of testing is important to ensure that issues can be resolved 'on-the-spot' and not be subject to interpretation after the event.

Their role is basically to:

- Provide advice as to whether a test may proceed when a test anomaly has been raised (see Section 8.13).

- Review a percentage of test results after the tests have been conducted (this percentage will have been defined as part of the Test Strategy). This is to ensure that results are adequately recorded and that the results justify the decision as to whether the test objective has been met and the test is a pass or fail.
- Provide advice as to the GxP impact of any test failure, proposed corrective actions and the scope of any retesting (see Section 8.15).

Regardless of whether or not someone from the Quality/Compliance function is available at the time, all test results and evidence should be of sufficient standard to allow later assessment of events to be made if required. However, having someone available at the time does reduce the risk of tests being continued when they should have been aborted or being aborted when they could continue.

### 8.6.6 Test Incident Manager

A person may be assigned to initially review and monitor all test incidents. This will include the categorisation of Test Incidents (see Section 8.14), the assessment of incidents and/or the assignment of Test Incidents for detailed assessment by others (see Section 8.15).

The Test Incident Manager should monitor the progress of all Test Incidents (often using a Test Incident Register) and should ensure that the overall Test Manager is kept up to date with regards to the status of the test incidents (also see Section 8.16).

## 8.7 Managing a Test Programme

The management of a large and complex Test Programme requires a Test Manager who is both an experienced tester and a good project manager. A good understanding of the technical issues involved is required, as is an ability to manage the interpersonal problems that can sometimes surface. The role involves:

- Assigning Testers and Test Witnesses to the execution of individual Test Scripts. This must be done in a way that makes best use of the available resource and respects the test order prerequisites (i.e. which tests must be conducted prior to others). Part of this process is an ability to predict how long an individual Test Script may take to execute. This becomes especially complex when tests have to be rerun and where it is more efficient to use the Tester who conducted the previous run (but may not be available, or may not be the best person to rerun a test due to 'tester errors' in the first run).
- Monitoring and reporting on the progress of the Test Programme. This can often be facilitated by the use of a computerised test management tool (see Section 8.16). This will often include keeping the overall Project Manager informed of progress and completion dates of various phases of the testing.
- Helping resolving any 'issues' between the Test team and the Quality/ Compliance organisation (who often see themselves with a different agenda).
- Balancing the need to meet test deadlines while still maintaining the integrity of the Test Programme. This is one of the hardest jobs to achieve. A good Test Manager will understand that it is better to deliver a properly tested system late than deliver a system that has not been properly tested on time.
- Ensuring that good test practice is observed throughout the Test Programme. This is achieved by monitoring the test statistics, liaison with the Quality/ Compliance organisation and by setting a good example with regard to tidiness, adherence to procedures, etc.

## 8.8 Checking Test Scripts In and Out

One of the most common problems is that of Test Scripts getting lost. It is embarrassing when any Test Script goes missing but doubly so when the Test Script has been executed and the loss of the test results requires the test to be conducted again.

There should be a process where all Test Scripts are signed out at the start of each test session and signed back in at the end of the session. In this way it will be known who is responsible for a Test Script at any given time. Test Scripts should be filed and secured between sessions.

All Test Script pages should be clearly identified (including any attachments) so that if they are mislaid and subsequently found, they can be returned to the correct Test Script. This should include the page number, the Test Script name or reference and the run number.

These problems can largely be overcome by the use of a computerised test management tool that automatically checks Test Scripts in and out.

## 8.9 Recording Test Results

It is a Regulatory expectation that Test Results are recorded quantitatively not qualitatively. In simple terms this means recording the actual value or number instead of just writing 'pass' or 'fail' or ticking a box.

The rationale behind this is to ensure that Test Results can be fully reviewed at a later date. If the actual result is recorded it is possible to review after the event whether the actual test objectives have been met.

This is of most critical concern for:

- Bespoke (customised) systems (GAMP software category 5)
- Highly GxP critical, GAMP category 4 or category 3 software
- Customised hardware (GAMP hardware category 2)

For these types of system, the quantitative recording of results should be treated as mandatory, especially during System Module Tests, Hardware Tests and Software Integration Tests. This does, however, impose an overhead on testing which may not be appropriate in all circumstances. In some cases it may be appropriate to make a qualitative record, for example, when:

- Separate evidence is provided (see Section 8.12) — this is applicable for all testing, although the test step should make clear reference to the evidence provided.
- The Test Script includes a clear range of acceptable results — this may be applicable for systems of low GxP criticality. In this case a mark should be made immediately alongside the stated range (i.e. ticking in a box alongside text stating '9.997 <= result<= 10.003', or 'displayed colour = red').
- The test step is not critical to proving that the test objective has been met (i.e. a set-up step). In these cases it is acceptable to provide a qualitative mark that the step has been executed (tick a box marked 'executed').
- The testing is part of a standard software test for a standard device (usually GAMP software category 2 and 3), with a clearly defined testing process.
- The testing is part of the normal manufacturing tests for standard hardware (GAMP hardware category 2).

In the latter two cases, where the test is conducted manually it is applicable to record a qualitative mark to indicate that a step has been executed and that the expected result is within a range clearly defined in the Test Script. Under these circumstances it is acceptable to write 'pass' (or tick a box marked 'pass' for each step).

For some automated manufacturing tests the quantitative value or the 'pass' or 'fail' qualitative status may be recorded automatically.

## 8.10 To Sign or Not to Sign

Should a Tester sign each step? This is one of the questions that the industry has been pondering for a long time. This is a mandatory requirement for testing in some healthcare companies but not in others.

This again imposes an overhead on testing and the question must be answered on a case-by-case basis by considering the following points:

- What is the GxP criticality of the test? Systems or functions with a low GxP criticality may justifiably demand a lower level of signed corroboration.
- What is the purpose of the step? If the step is required in order to set up the system for subsequent steps that actually demonstrate the test objective, a signature may not be required for the set up step or steps. This is especially the case where the correct set-up is clearly demonstrated by evidence such as a screen shot or where a witness observes the set-up prior to executing the key step.

Where there is doubt about the requirement to provide a full signature, a step may be initialled as a compromise measure.

Regardless of which steps are signed (or initialled) by the tester, the completed test must always be signed off and the context of the signature must always be clear. An example of such a statement could be:

'Signed to confirm that all of the above test steps were conducted in a contiguous manner, in accordance with the test instructions for each step and that the recorded results are an accurate record of the test execution'.

The Test Script should also include a clear statement of whether the test objective was met or not and whether the test was passed.

## 8.11 The Use of Test Witnesses

Given the potential GxP impact of testing, it is important that test results cannot be falsified. To meet the expectations of certain of the Regulatory authorities this includes taking adequate steps to ensure that test records cannot be falsified.

This may be achieved by attaching test evidence (see Section 8.12) or by the use of Test Witnesses. The use of Test Witnesses should be decided upon on a pragmatic basis since the use of a witness adds to the cost of testing and often slows down the testing process.

The guiding principle should be that for GxP critical tests, where no adequate proof of testing can be obtained by other means (see Section 8.12), a Test Witness will be required to ensure that the Test Objective has been met (see Section 8.11).

For some tests this may require that the witness observes every step. This is likely where the test is designed to demonstrate a sequence of events, such as a functional work flow. In this case the witness must observe every step. Signing each step is not mandatory so long as the Witness signs at the completion of the test. This signature should include a statement that the context of the signature is such that the Witness has observed every step and concurs that the recorded results and/or evidence and any comments or notes that the Tester has made are an accurate record of the test run. Unless such a statement is included, it will be necessary for the Witness to sign every step.

For other tests, where the initial test steps are only required to set up data or to place the system in a specific state to prove the test objective, it may not be necessary for the Witness to observe all of the preliminary set-up steps. In this case the Witness may observe and sign at the specific test step that proves the test objective or may sign at the completion of the test, with a suitable statement as to the context of the signature.

A Test Witness must always understand what he/she is observing and must understand the objective of the test. This may require adequate knowledge of the system or application under test and may require prior training or briefing.

If a Test Witness does not understand the purpose of the test or any specific step, he/she should seek clarification before that test or step proceeds. If he/she is not happy that he/she has understood the objective of the test, if he/she is unsure whether the test objective has been met, or if he/she believes that the test was not properly conducted, he/she should either refuse to sign or more properly raise a Test Anomaly to review the situation.

The use of Test Witnesses may also be required for contractual reasons, where a User wishes to ensure that the Functional Testing does adequately prove that the system meets its business needs.

## 8.12 Capturing Test Evidence (Raw Data)

It is sometimes easier to capture test evidence than to record such evidence by hand. This test evidence may be produced by:

- An automated test system or test software, which produces a summary report of the test steps, input and output data
- Reports or other output produced as part of a test
- Screen shots of screen data or status

All test evidence should be securely attached to the completed Test Script. Reference should be made to the associated test evidence at the appropriate step in the Test (in a comments column or a column specially included to refer to attached evidence).

The creative 'design' of screen shots can be used to record a good deal of evidence that minimises the need for adding additional data manually. Using standard display 'windows' it is often possible to compose a screen shot that contains the date and time, the actual evidence in the form of one or more applications windows and even additional data such as the ID or network address (IP address, MAC address, etc.) of the workstation the test was conducted on.

When computerised test tools are used the screen shot can be captured electronically and pasted into a document, which can be electronically linked to the executed Test Script, thereby doing away with any paper evidence.

For standard manufacturing test reports it is acceptable to sign these and file them without the report being attached to a specific Test Script.

Depending upon the data contained in the output it may be necessary to manually annotate the evidence with details such as date/time, serial number of unit under test, test run number, number of pages, etc. When designing such tests it is always useful to include such data in the report header.

## 8.13 Proceed or Abort? (Test Incident Management)

If Test Script instructions are not clearly written or if the system under test behaves in an unexpected manner, it is sometimes difficult for an inexperienced tester to know what to do.

They may choose to continue to execute a test to completion when the test should have been aborted. This may waste minutes, hours or even days conducting a test that may have to be performed again.

In other cases they may abort a test when that test could have been continued through to completion. This may be because the language used in the instructions is not clear to the Tester or if a system dialogue box contains a message that is slightly different to the 'expected result'. If this occurs towards the end of a test it can again waste a great deal of time.

If the Tester (or Witness) is in any doubt they should always seek advice from the Lead Tester, possibly the Test Incident Manager or the Quality/Compliance representative. This can be raised as an anomaly and investigated informally.

Where the anomaly is minor (a typographical error on the Test Script) and the intent of the test and the result is reasonably clear, it may be possible to continue the test and raise a Change Note to revise the Test Script. The justification for this should be recorded as a comment on the completed Test Script and signed and dated by those involved in resolving the anomaly.

If the resolution is not immediate there are two options:

- Record the anomaly as a Test Incident and continue the test to completion, in the anticipation that the anomaly can be resolved and the results of the test will still be valid.
- Abort the test and raise a Test Incident.

It should be noted that if two or three anomalies are recorded during a Test Script execution the outcome of the test would be very difficult to evaluate and justify after the event. A test should usually be stopped once a second anomaly has occurred.

Note also that Test Scripts should be reviewed for recorded anomalies. A trend may indicate a problem with either a specific Tester or the author of specific Test Scripts and a need for retraining may be indicated.

## 8.14 Categorising Test Incidents

If a test is aborted a Test Incident should be raised. This can also be raised in the case of an anomaly that cannot be immediately resolved.

All Test Incidents should be assessed and part of this assessment process includes assigning a Test Incident Category. Tests Incidents can be categorised as follows:

- Test Script error – there is an error in the Test Script which caused the test to fail, or which means that either the instructions were not clear, or could not be executed.
- Tester Error – the error was as a result of the Tester either making a mistake (mis-keying data) or not understanding clear instructions or results.
- Set-up Error – the test set up was incorrectly performed causing the test to fail or meaning that the test execution could not continue.
- Test Data Error – there was an error in the test dataset(s), causing the test to fail or meaning that the test execution could not continue.
- External Failure – there was an unforeseen external event such as a power failure, causing the test to fail, or meaning that the test execution could not continue.
- Configuration Error – there was a problem with the configuration of the system under test, causing the test to fail or meaning that the test execution could not continue.

- Application Error – there is a fault with the software under test, causing the test to failor meaning that the test execution could not continue.
- Procedural Failure – there was a problem with an operating procedure that was being followed as part of the test, which caused the test to fail or which meant that the test execution could not continue.

Note that this list is not exhaustive and that other categories may be defined depending upon the nature of the system under test.

An analysis of the Test Incident Categories will provide an indication of the validity and value of the testing programme. If most of the Test Incidents are as a result of configuration, application or procedural errors then this demonstrates the validity of the testing by finding such errors.

If most of the problems are due to Test Script errors, set-up errors, Tester errors or test data errors this calls into question the validity of the testing. During a Test Programme the number of such errors should decrease over time. If an upward trend is detected, or if the number of such errors exceeds 40% after the first week of testing, a halt should be called to testing. This may require Test Scripts and datasets to be reviewed again or Testers to be retrained.

Computerised test management tools allow such categories to be assigned to Test Incidents and statistical data generated.

Note that the capture and analysis of test performance data is one of the key components in defining and rationalising a risk-based approach to testing (see Section 3.3).

## 8.15 Impact Assessment

All Test Incidents must be assessed. If there is any doubt as to the GxP impact of the incident, this assessment should include a representative of the Quality or Compliance department. In some organisations a representative of the Compliance department will review and assess all Test Incidents. This may not be necessary where the Test Incident Manager has a sufficient degree of regulatory awareness to decide whether or not to involve the Compliance representative.

The impact assessment must determine:

- Whether or not the test must be repeated (in the case of an anomaly raised as an Incident during Test Script execution).
- Changes that will have to be made to correct the error.
- The extent of any re-testing that will be required as a result of the changes made. Note that this assessment is greatly facilitated by using Configuration Management records to determine the interrelationships between the changed items and any other configuration items.

There must be a formal process for managing Test Incidents. This must define the stages that an Incident will go through (typically raised, initial assessment, allocation (to a person for detailed assessment), detailed assessment, approval to fix, fix, approval to close and closed — see Section 8.6 for a typical Incident life cycle). This must also define the roles and responsibilities of those involved in managing the Test Incident.

Note that the 'fix' may just require the raising of a Change Note and once this has been done the Incident may be closed. Alternatively, changes may be made under the governance of a Test Incident (following an approved Test Incident Procedure), so long as all changes are referenced to the Test Incident.

## 8.16 Test Execution Status

In order to monitor the progress of the Test Programme, it is useful to have an overview of the test execution status. Figures can be maintained manually or a good computerised test management tool will provide statistics such as:

- Total number of Test Scripts
- Number of Test Scripts not executed (and as a percentage of the total)
- Number of Test Scripts passed (also as a %)
- Number of Test Scripts passed first run (also as a % of the total and as a % of the total passed)
- Average number of Test Runs per Test Script
- Etc.

These statistics are useful for not just monitoring the progress of the Test Programme, but of the validity and value of the Test Programme. If a low number of Test Scripts are being passed first time, or if the average number of Test Runs per Test Scripts is more than 2, this may indicate a problem with the testing. The Test Incident Category statistics should be reviewed to determine the cause of the problem (see Section 7.14).

## 8.17 Test Data Status

Where simple numerical calculations are tested it is relatively easy to define test datasets with pre-defined input criteria. These can be referenced by a number of tests.

In some complex systems the use of system test data requires significant thought. Where a test modifies a data object in such a way that it cannot be changed back again (i.e. a document is moved from 'draft' to 'reviewed' status or a batch is changed from 'quarantined' to 'released') that data object cannot be used for the same test. This is because the Test Script assumes that the data object is in its initial state, which is no longer the case.

This is often made more complex when several tests may be using the same data object. As an example, one test could change a document from 'draft' to 'reviewed' and a different test changes it from 'reviewed' to 'draft'. This is even more complicated where the object does not follow a known sequence of states but can be changed from any state to any state.

This is not a problem when Tests Scripts pass first time but if they fail and have to be rerun the test data objects many be in the wrong status to repeat the test.

In these cases the management of test data objects needs careful consideration and some solutions might be:

- Sequence tests so that they use test data objects in the status they have been left in by previously executed tests. This is only likely to work in small or simple systems with a limited number of tests.
- Define groups of test data objects that can be independently saved and restored prior to tests being executed. The reload of such data object sets would be part of the set-up for each test. This is only practical in systems which allow partial data object sets to be saved and restored.
- Write the Test Script in such a way as to use any suitable data object that is in the necessary state to conduct the test. In this case the name of the object would have to be recorded as part of the Test Script execution, and any expected results would have to refer to the recorded object name rather than a fixed object name. This then allows any suitable data object to be used (or created).

### 8.18 Test Log-On Accounts (User IDs)

Clarity of login accounts is crucial when testing systems with defined user profiles.

It is important that actions taken as a Tester and actions taken as a User are clearly differentiated.

Specific user accounts should be created for the purposes of testing and these should be granted appropriate privileges or assigned appropriate user profiles for the functions under test. The allocation and use of these for testing should be recorded. These user IDs should be created and maintained using appropriate user authorisation procedures. This tests not only the profile-based functionality of the system but also the user authorisation processes as well as the user management functions within the system.

These login IDs should be used to execute tests. This is to ensure that profiles with appropriate permissions are used to test the functionality and security of the system. Once testing is complete these User ID's access rights should be removed from the system, although a record of the User IDs should be maintained to ensure their uniqueness within the system (i.e. to ensure that a duplicate ID is not assigned in the future).

Where Testers have their own user IDs these should not be used for testing user functionality. This is because a Tester may have an inappropriate profile for the test. Where a Tester has to reconfigure the functionality of the system as part of the test, this should be done using their individual User ID (to differentiate actions conducted as part of the test script execution using a defined user profile, and those conducted external to the test script execution as a tester).

There should be no group log-ins for the system and any Tester's actions should be directly attributable to them individually. Where it is necessary to modify any user's authority or permissions this should be done using the appropriate system access and authorisation procedures.

Test Scripts should explicitly state the login ID to use during testing. Instructions such as 'login to the system' are ambiguous and should read 'log-in to the system as user 'gdg_tester_1'.

CHAPTER 9

# Supplier System Test Reports/Qualification Reports

Depending upon the nature of the testing, it may be usual for suppliers to produce System Test Reports that summarise the results of the System Testing.

Depending upon the size and complexity of the testing, this may:

- Be incorporated into a single report, detailing all of the system testing. This is most appropriate for small or simple systems.
- Require a separate Test Summary Report for each level of testing (i.e. Hardware Test Summary Report, Software Module Test Summary Report).

Such Test Summary Reports should include an overview of the test results and may include statistical data such as:

- Total number of tests executed
- Percentage passed first time
- Total number of test reruns

This should also include a list of any critical test non-compliances and any outstanding issues that remain, such as system functions that have not satisfactorily completed Acceptance Testing.

The report should include a clear indication of whether or not subsequent phases of testing may proceed with justifications as to why.

Where the supplier does not produce such reports, this should be included in the relevant Qualification Report (IQ, OQ or PQ Report, depending upon the level of testing). Where the supplier does provide such reports, they should be referenced in the relevant Qualification Report, thereby reducing unnecessary duplication.

Where the Test Report or summary only relates to a single test, or series of tests, it is often useful to attach the actual test record sheets to the back of the Report. This makes it much easier to reference the detail recorded in the actual test sheets.

CHAPTER 10

# The Use of Electronic Test Management and Automated Test Tools

## 10.1 The Need for Test Tools in the Pharmaceutical Industry

The Healthcare Industries have a need to reduce the cost of implementing IT systems and solutions. This is even more important than in other industries because of the relatively high price it pays for testing its computer systems in a highly regulated environment.

The use of computer based test management and automated test tools ('computerised test tools') can reduce the time taken to develop and execute Test Scripts and can significantly reduce the number of human errors. These cost savings are accrued by the faster development and execution of Test Scripts. Significant savings also result from the reduced number of test execution errors and the resulting reduction in the need to analyse incidents and repeat tests due to human error.

In addition to the cost savings available, the reduced number of test execution errors and the ability to easily trace Test Scripts to individual Requirements helps build a strong validation case. It is not uncommon for well-specified and well-designed systems to have their quality (and subsequent validation status) badly compromised by a poor set of Test Scripts and test results. The use of an automated test tool can greatly improve the control of Test Scripts and reduce the number of test execution errors.

A more significant benefit can also be obtained when systems are being changed or upgraded. This is especially the case in large or complex systems where many software patches may need to be applied and the inter-relationship of these 'patches' makes it very difficult to rationally define the scope of any retesting. This is because not even the software developers can track all the interdependencies in their complex software packages. In these cases, the only safe solution is to retest the entire system, as appropriate to the GxP risk (justified in the original Test Strategy).

The ability to quickly and easily repeat tests (for instance, user profile/security tests) using automated Test Scripts means that upgrades are significantly faster and less expensive to implement. This in turn means that the advantages of changes and upgrades are much more likely to be fully realised and that the validated status is much more likely to be adequately maintained.

The use of computerised test tools therefore offers significant cost savings and improved support for validating computer systems and is of benefit to most pharmaceutical manufacturers and healthcare companies.

## 10.2 Test Tool Functionality

Computerised test tools basically provide three useful features, namely:

- The ability to manage Test Scripts and Test Incidents in an electronic (paperless) environment while still executing the Test Scripts manually. Such systems also provide the tools to plan test campaigns and report on the status of the test campaign, analyse test results, allocate Test Scripts to Test Engineers and so on.
- The ability to automatically execute Test Scripts, including the recording of Test Results. Most test tool systems in widespread use have standard interfaces to the most popular system interfaces and have the ability to interact with standard user interfaces written using standard technologies such as JavaScript, ActiveX controls, Visual Basic, etc.
- The ability to 'load test' a system, by simulating the load of many hundreds of simultaneous users. The ability to repeat such tests is a useful aid to on-going performance monitoring of systems.

### 10.3 Electronic Records and Electronic Signature Compliance

Despite the obvious benefits to be gained from using such systems, they are not in widespread use for testing GxP critical systems. There are two main reasons for this.

Firstly, as described above, such systems can provide significant cost savings and have an attractive payback period. However, the purchase, implementation, rollout and validation costs of such test tools are still significant. In order to achieve the anticipated cost savings and payback it is necessary to initially use the automated test tool in support of a significant IT project. Examples of this are large ERP systems, the development of standard products such as Clinical Trial Management systems or global Intranet, Extranet and Internet applications.

The other reason for not adopting such systems has been the lack of regulatory compliance (test record integrity) required when testing GxP critical systems in the Healthcare Industries. In order to sell pharmaceutical products, biological products or medical devices into various markets the safety of such products must be assured. This is facilitated by various Regulatory agencies (the FDA, MHRA, etc) that enforce various legislation, standards and guidelines in a number of areas.

So called 'Predicate Rules' deal with issues directly impacting and controlling Good Clinical, Laboratory, Manufacturing or Distribution Practice. Examples of these are Chapter 21 of the US Code of Federal Regulations, Parts 210, 211, 606 and 820, EU Directive 91/356/EEC, etc.

The Predicate Rules are supported by additional regulations and guidelines that deal with issues which may directly or indirectly affect product quality, data integrity (and possibly patient safety). This includes the use of computer systems for the design, manufacture, testing and distribution of such products and devices and is directly governed by regulations such as 21CFR Part 11, Part 211.68, Part 820, 91/356/EEC Annex 11 and so on.

Inherent with these regulations is the use of records and signatures used to support GxP critical processes. Various computer systems support or control processes that are covered under the Predicate Rules and such systems are clearly GxP critical. In addition, the testing of such systems is also covered under supporting regulations. Any system that is used to test a GxP critical system is, therefore, also considered to be GxP critical (if only indirectly) and whilst test records are considered to be GxP critical records, they are not specifically mentioned in the majority of the predicate rules. Such test records are therefore not usually subject to the controls of 21CFR Part 11, but the integrity of such records does need to be assured in support of the validation of GxP critical systems.

If an automated test tool is used to test a computer system that supports a process covered under the Predicate Rules such a system must have adequate security around the approval, execution, post execution and long term storage of such testing records.

Most large computer systems which would economically justify the use of an automated test tool are GxP critical (at least in part) and any pharmaceutical manufacturer looking to use an automated test tool should be looking for a tool which can assure the integrity of test records (possibly supported by full audit trails and the use of electronic signatures).

## 10.4 The Availability of Suitable Test Tools

The developers of test tool applications were slow to realise the need to comply with industry requirements for test record integrity and the result is that test tools that can assure test record integrity are only just appearing on the market.

Even now, the choice of test tools that can be used in a compliant manner is extremely limited, with only one mainstream manufacturer having considered the specific requirements for test record integrity. It is expected that a number of other compliant solutions will appear on the market in the next few years, widening the choice for healthcare companies wishing to use such systems.

## 10.5 Test Script Life Cycle

The advantages of using an automated test tool for Test Script management are largely around the processes ('workflow') associated with Test Script authoring, reviewing, approval, execution and post execution review and approval (Figure 10.1).

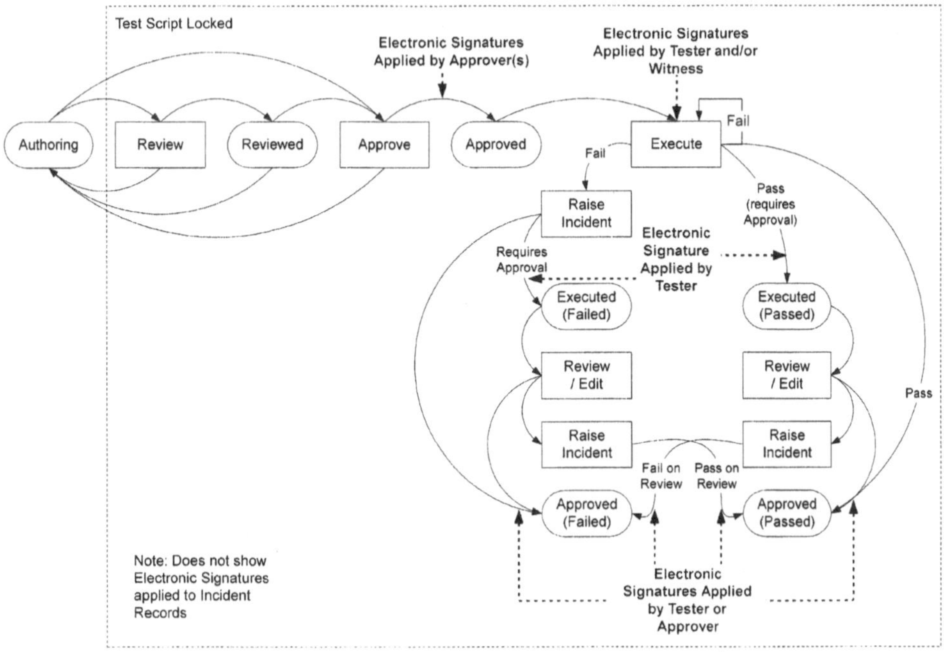


**Figure 10.1 – The Test Script Life Cycle.**

Performing the testing in an automated, paperless environment allows it to be done in a more efficient and more controlled manner, across one or more sites. This is especially useful when

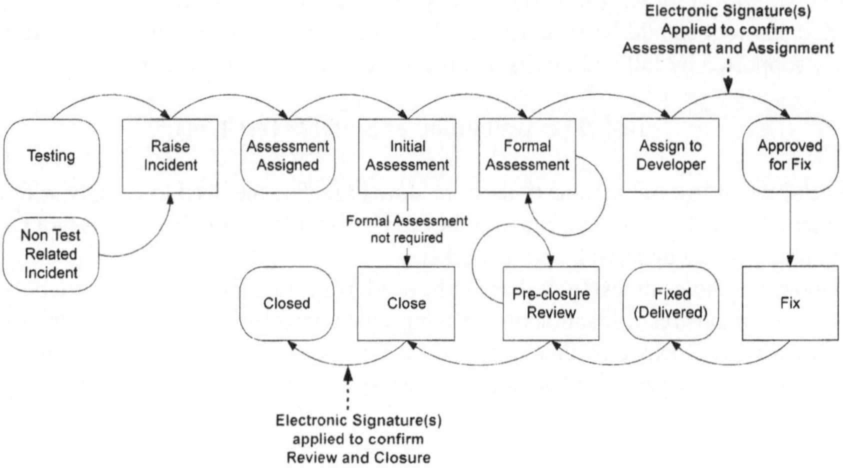


**Figure 10.2 – The Test Incident Life Cycle.**

the development and execution of Test Scripts is conducted by a team based on several sites or, possibly, in different countries.

One useful feature that such systems support is the ability to enter which User or Functional Requirements are tested by each Test Script. This helps to ensure that complete test coverage is achieved (untested Requirements can be highlighted).

In order to meet the requirements for test record integrity Test Script may be treated as an electronic record. Approval and execution signatures may be treated as electronic signatures, and there should be adequate proof of a formal review (note that this is suggested, and is not mandated by most predicate rules).

Defining the 'Test Script Life Cycle' allows changes in the electronic record status and points at which electronic signatures are applied to be clearly defined. This approach also facilitates the determination of 'who can do what and when', which in turn makes it easier to define user profiles (e.g. Test Script Author, Test Witness, Test Run Approver, etc.). This ensures that only persons with defined access rights and privileges can perform various review, approval and execution tasks.

## 10.6 Incident Life Cycle

In a similar way to Test Scripts, a life cycle approach can also be taken for Incident Management (Figure 10.2). This will define the changes in status for an Incident (e.g. open, assessed, approved, implemented, closed), where electronic signatures may be used and who is allowed to sign (again based upon user profiles).

Unlike Test Scripts, Incidents have no 'draft' status – as soon as an Incident is raised it is subject to formal management.

An efficient system should allow Test Script details to be passed directly to an Incident Record (i.e. Test Script name and reference, step and run number, Requirements reference, tester ID, etc.). It should also allow non-test related ('ad-hoc') Incidents to be raised and managed.

A good computerised test tools system will allow a flexible life cycle to be applied to individual projects, or even individual Test Scripts. This is useful for GxP risk-based testing where the standard of compliance or quality review may be higher or lower than other areas, based upon the principle defined in the Test Approaches and Test Strategy.

### 10.7 Flexibility for Non-GxP Use

In order to be most useful to Life Science companies, a computerised test tool should be capable of supporting the testing of both GxP and non-GxP systems.

The testing of GxP systems imposes additional requirements in order to comply with specific regulatory requirements and expectations. Examples of these are the need to capture proof of test objectives being met (by electronically attaching screen copies for instance), the need for witness signatures or the need for post execution review and approval.

Some of these are an unnecessary overhead when testing non-GxP systems. A cost effective automated test tool should allow these additional requirements to be turned off when used to test non-GxP systems.

However, when testing GxP critical systems it must be impossible for the user to bypass these requirements (see Section 10.10).

### 10.8 Project and Compliance Approach

The selection, procurement, development, integration, testing and validation of a computerised test tool is different from that of other computer based systems. This is because GAMP 4 defines a 'Tools' category for certain types of system that support the implementation of GxP critical systems or GxP functions.

A computerised test tool is not as critical as a manufacturing system that packages tablets or sterilises medical devices. It is arguably less critical than a system that maintains training records for individuals performing GxP critical processes against controlled procedures.

Because a computerised Test Tool does not have a direct impact on product quality or identity (and thereby has no direct impact on patient safety) it does not require stringent validation. However, if the system is not secure, the integrity of test records may be called into doubt, because of the possibility of accidentally modifying or deliberately falsifying test records.

A computerised test tool should therefore be validated but the Validation Plan should assume that this is a system with low GxP criticality.

### 10.9 Testing Test Tools

The approach to testing a computerised test tool should be to treat it as a development tool. Where the tool is in widespread use in the Healthcare Industries testing may be limited to Functional Testing only. If the system is not in widespread use in the Healthcare Industry, challenge testing will be required to demonstrate the integrity of the Test Scripts, Test Incidents and Test Results. This challenge testing should specifically demonstrate that the system is secure.

Good practice would suggest that a system that has not been tested should not be used in operation, which infers that an automated test tool should not be used to test itself, at least, not for an initial rollout. This means that an automated test tool should be tested manually in the first instance. Consequently, testing the system is prone to the potential problems that the system is designed to replace — there is nothing that can be done about this except encouraging and enforcing 'Good Testing Practice'.

The life cycles defined in the development of the system can also be used as the basis for developing manual test procedures and the necessary Test Scripts and Incident Management processes and forms. The same life cycles can be used to manage the Test Scripts and Test

Incidents, albeit in a paper based environment. This will help to demonstrate the validity of the defined life cycles.

Testing an automated test tool brings additional complications because of the terminology. Clear definitions are required in order to avoid confusion around statements such as '…the objective of this Test Script is to test the Test Script Approval process…'. The potential adverse impact of this cannot be overstated (nor the potential for finding humour in the testing of a test system).

If the computerised test tool has been customised, the system will need more comprehensive testing. Such testing will include Software Module Testing. Additional negative testing or stress testing should focus on areas of bespoke functional development (such as user profile testing, audit trail testing, etc.) and the stress testing of the infrastructure.

## 10.10 Test Record Integrity

Any computerised test tool must be secure. As well as assuring basic test record integrity and assuring that users cannot readily repudiate any electronic signatures, these security requirements also include the need to:

- Archive test records and test record audit trails, in line with the users record retention policy
- Ensure that user editable 'on-line' system documentation (i.e. help files, electronic user manuals, etc.) are managed as secure files

As stated above, there are currently very few automated test tools that are capable of meeting such security requirements and even these systems will need additional procedural controls to be put in place.

A good computerised test tool will provide support for the procedural controls. These include:

- The ability to produce lists of users and their assigned user profiles, so that these may be reviewed on a regular basis.
- The ability to require users to change their passwords on a regular basis, to define minimum length passwords and the ability to prevent the re-use of recently used passwords.
- The ability to support a proceduralised approach to granting user access on a 'need to do' (user profile) basis.
- An ability to manage users' system specific training records, including revoking access rights when retraining is required.

It should be noted that the list of technical and procedural requirements stated above are far from comprehensive and need to be reviewed with respect to current regulations and guidance.

## 10.11 Features to Look Out For

Based upon the above, any healthcare company looking to purchase a computerised test tool should base their decision upon the following criteria:

- A proven track record of supplying such tools to the Healthcare Industries
- An ability to manage Test Scripts and Test Incidents in a paperless environment
- The ability to support traceability between User Requirements, Specifications and individual Test Scripts or Tests

- The ability to automatically execute Test Scripts
- The ability to support a wide variety of system user interfaces
- The ability to perform load and volume testing
- The flexibility to efficiently test non-GxP systems, by 'turning off' the electronic records audit trail and electronic signature capability on a project-by-project basis

CHAPTER 11

# Appendix A – Hardware Test Specification and Testing

## 11.1 Defining the Hardware Test Strategy

Assuming that Hardware Category 1 hardware is genuinely standard hardware in widespread use, specific testing of the hardware is not required. For Category 1 hardware it is sufficient to demonstrate that the hardware has been manufactured in accordance with the requirements of a recognised quality system (e.g. ISO 9000).

Where available, standard manufacturer's test records may be used to support the validation case for systems of medium or high GxP Criticality. Specific hardware acceptance testing is not required since this will be implicitly tested as part of the System Acceptance Testing.

In cases where the hardware is Category 2 (customised), system specific testing will be required and this may also be the case if Category 1 hardware is used outside the operating conditions specified by the manufacturer.

The degree of testing of Category 2 hardware should be applicable to the GxP Criticality of the system being tested. For example, it may be sufficient to test systems of low GxP Criticality within the normal operating range, without testing outside the range, if there is a low probability of this range being exceeded in operation.

For systems of high GxP Criticality it may be justified to test outside this range in order that failure modes may be predicted and contingency plans made. Further examples of this are discussed below.

It should also be noted that many systems that have some degree of customisation will also contain many standard system components and that the Test Strategy would need to distinguish between the two.

The objectives of the Hardware Tests should be clearly traceable to the appropriate sections of the Hardware Specification. Meeting the objectives of the Package Configuration Test Scripts should clearly demonstrate that the hardware is built and operates as specified.

Issues to consider for Hardware Testing follow.

## 11.2 Standard Test Methods

There are many different methods of conducting standard Hardware Acceptance Tests and these vary according to system type and from manufacturer to manufacturer.

Each 'method' will define a series of steps, conducted in a repeatable sequence in order to demonstrate that the objectives of the test(s) are met.

It is likely that different test methods will be used for different types of test. For example, the correct functioning of a standard printed circuit board can be tested using Automated Test Equipment (ATE). Individual component parts may also be subject to Functional Testing such as heat-soak tests and burn-in tests. These are usually part of standard manufacturing tests.

Other tests may be project specific and may require particular input conditions to be physically created, simulated or manually entered.

Tests may be conducted using a combination of standard or specific test methods that provide the appropriate challenges to verify hardware operation and performance.

Modern day hardware is often controlled by firmware. Such firmware provides control functions that assure that the hardware components deliver the stated functionality. Tests on firmware-controlled hardware must take into consideration GAMP validation categories.

A number of example test methods are described below. Specific test methods will be described in the actual Hardware Acceptance Test Specification, either in the General section or in the individual sections of the Hardware Acceptance Test Specification.

The detail in which the test is described may vary according to the general test methodology described in the General section of the Hardware Acceptance Test Specification. It may be necessary to provide detailed step-by-step instructions (including providing full details of set-up instruction or individual keystrokes for the test engineer to follow) or it may be acceptable to provide general instructions that rely on the test engineer using an overall knowledge of the hardware system under test.

Where the test method requires prerequisite knowledge of the hardware it should be clearly stated in the General section of the Hardware Acceptance Test Specification.

Wherever possible, general test methods should be used and documented in the General section of the Hardware Acceptance Test Specification. In this case it is acceptable for the individual section of the Hardware Acceptance Test Specification to reference a General section of the Hardware Acceptance Test Specifications. For example '*Select channel 1 on analogue input card AI13 and set the input value to 4mA — refer to Section 1.2 of test procedure "Testing Current Input Modules" for specific instructions*'.

When defining the test methods to be used the following issues must be considered.

## 11.3 Manual Testing of Component Hardware

In some circumstances, printed circuit cards, populated printed circuit boards and system components (electrical or mechanical) may be subject to manual testing and this will usually be part of the manufacturer's standard Quality Assurance procedures.

Manual tests may vary but usually include the use of equipment such as logic probes, multimeters, customised test rigs, etc.

Systems should be in place in order to ensure that:

- Documentary evidence of the individual board or item under test (including art work revision number, firmware version number, drawing number and serial number) is generated
- The test rig the test was performed on is referenced
- Testers details are recorded
- The name and version number of the test procedure used is documented
- The date and time of the test is recorded
- The test results are clear and accurate
- Details of any failure are documented

### 11.3.1 Automated Test Equipment

A large proportion of testing of unpopulated printed circuit cards and populated printed circuit boards is conducted using Automated Test Equipment (ATE). This is usually part of the manufacturer's standard Quality Assurance programme and has the advantage of being thorough and efficient.

These systems can provide sufficient evidence of testing so long as supporting systems are in place to provide:

- Documentary evidence of the individual board under test (including art work revision number, firmware version number and serial number)
- The ATE machine the test was performed on
- The ATE test jig used (including drawing revision or version number)
- The revision of the ATE Test Programme being run
- The date and time of the test
- The test results
- Details of any failure

Supplier audits should challenge the tests conducted using ATEs. Tests should sufficiently test operating limits to ensure that the board is thoroughly tested, not only for 'correct operation' but also for items which could lead to subsequent failure, such as 'dry joints', short circuits, etc.

Should any individual board fail ATE testing, a system should be in place to record the details of the fault, any rework and subsequent re-testing as described above for manual testing. A maximum number of retests should also be defined before a card or board is scrapped as unusable (before the cost of retesting and rework outweighs the value of the board).

### 11.3.2 Burn-In/Heat Soak Tests

Burn-in tests are often conducted to identify circuit boards that may pass a detailed test, but still may be likely to premature failure due to manufacturing defects or individual component failures.

Such tests are again likely to be part of the manufacturer's standard Quality Assurance procedures. These tests should provide documentary evidence of:

- The boards or items under test (including art work revision number, firmware version number and serial number)
- The equipment the test was performed on
- The revision of the Test Programme being run (a good burn-in test will usually sequence through a series of temperature changes, possibly including a 'heat soak' test at elevated temperature)
- The date and time of the test
- The test results
- Details of any failure(s)

The manufacturer should again have a system to record the details of any fault(s), any rework and subsequent retesting following the heat soak test (for instance, how many failures will be allowed? Will ATE testing be required again before another heat soak test? etc.).

### 11.3.3 Standard Integrated Hardware Tests

Testing of integrated hardware components is essential to ensure that they collectively meet performance requirements and that hardware event synchronisation functions correctly.

These tests may, for instance, test such basic functions as:

- Network communication

- Field communication
- Data storage and retrieval
- System performance under normal and maximum loading
- Error handling and recovery (including power outages)

The following information must be recorded:

- Documentary evidence of the component hardware items under test (usually just serial number at this stage)
- Details of any support equipment used for the test
- The revision number of the test procedure being tested
- The date and time of the test
- The test results
- Details of any failure(s)

These tests are very important where standard hardware is being used in a non-standard configuration or architecture and systems of medium or high GxP Criticality should 'stress test' points at which the hardware is integrated to ensure that interfaces are predictable and robust. This is even more important where custom hardware from different manufacturers has been integrated into a complete system.

This may also be useful for medium or high GxP Critical systems when standard hardware (Hardware Category 1) from different manufacturers is integrated in a non-standard or unusual manner. As a minimum, the compatibility of such components may be verified by comparing equipment specifications, written confirmation from suppliers, etc.

### 11.3.4 Automated Testing

Conducting the Hardware Acceptance Tests can be a time consuming and expensive process given the need to fully test every component piece of hardware. This task can be eased by the use of automated testing and most manufacturers have invested in this technology to reduce their manufacturing and QA costs.

Automated testing combines the functions of simulation and automatic data recording to fully automate the task of hardware testing. Such facilities lend themselves to the testing of many similar hardware devices and can either conduct a single test at a time or can conduct many tests in sequence or parallel.

Automated testing is likely to be part of the standard manufacturing tests but if it is necessary to develop project specific automated testing applications these should be controlled and reviewed as part of the Hardware Acceptance Test Specification.

### 11.3.5 Hardware Acceptance Test Methods

The system hardware is an essential part of a complete validated solution and correctly conducted and documented Hardware Acceptance Tests are an integral part of the validation documentation set.

Hardware is implicitly tested as part of a System Acceptance Test and standard hardware (Hardware Category 1) does not require hardware acceptance testing. Where the hardware is customised (Hardware Category 2) hardware acceptance testing is required.

The nature and extent of hardware acceptance testing must be applicable to the GxP Priority of the system. Where it is possible to segregate hardware into different levels of GxP Priority (which is usually only possible for certain types of manufacturing, control or automation systems) different hardware components may be subject to different levels of testing.

As a minimum, Hardware Acceptance Tests must test the correct operation of the hardware across the full operating range. For systems of medium or high GxP Priority it is also useful to test the system outside the normal operating range in order to predict what may or will happen (the 'failure mode'). Specific emphasis must be placed on the areas of customisation.

An example of why this is necessary could be a customised control system, the individual components of which are designed to operate between 0 and 50°C. The actual environment in which it is installed may be controlled to between 18 and 25°C but if the HVAC system fails, what is the minimum and maximum temperature that may be reached? If the temperature were likely to exceed 50°C (in certain enclosed areas of a production line for instance) what would the effect be on the customised system? If the customised hardware repeatedly fails in a catastrophic and unpredictable manner at just 42°C, it may be necessary to require that all manufacturing operations cease if the HVAC system fails. If the system monitors ambient temperature and performs an orderly shutdown at 50°C, with no critical data being lost, it may be possible to state that manufacturing operations may continue up to 45°C, subject to on-going temperature monitoring. All of the above assumes that no personnel work in the area and that the product is not subject to any adverse effects in such conditions.

When determining the extent of such tests it is, therefore, necessary to understand the nature of the customisation and the associated risks, the GxP Criticality of the system (or function) and the expected failure mode.

The complexity of such testing highlights the fact that standard (Category 1) hardware should be used wherever possible.

Careful consideration must be given to the use of standard test methodologies, efficient test sequencing, appropriate control and utilisation of tools, equipment and personnel.

## 11.4 Performance Baseline

In order to ensure that meaningful performance monitoring may be conducted during the operational phase of the system, it is useful to establish a hardware performance baseline during hardware testing.

This would include taking hardware performance measurements (or capturing records) under controlled conditions that could also be established during the operation of the system. These may include:

- The number of hardware (device) errors over a specified period of time
- Signal/noise ratio measurements
- Verification of screen display clarity (under known light conditions, at defined distances, etc.)
- Number of network errors and retries with a known data loading

It is useful to measure performance in a known 'clean' environment so that any problems with the system hardware can be distinguished from installation problems. This baseline can be established as part of the FAT and repeated as part of the SAT.

This is especially useful with performance that may degrade over time, such as system grounding (earthing), screen degradation, etc.

CHAPTER 12

# Appendix B – Package Configuration Test Specifications and Testing

## 12.1 Defining the Package Configuration Test Strategy

The overall combination of Package Configuration Verification, Functional Testing and stress testing needs to be appropriate to:

- The GxP Criticality
- Any prior experience with the package (that is documented)
- The size and complexity of the overall system

The level and nature of verification/testing of each package will be unique to each system, should be well thought out by experienced personnel and documented and justified as part of the Test Strategy.

The objectives of the Package Configuration Tests should be clearly traceable to the appropriate sections of the Package Configuration Specification. Meeting the objectives of the Package Configuration Test Scripts should clearly demonstrate that the system is configured as specified.

## 12.2 Configurable Systems

Many software applications require a number of 'configuration' settings to be made. These involve the setting of various parameters that determine how the system (or software module) will function.

The setting of these parameters may involve:

- The entry of numerical settings in a field (such as a constant, a multiplication factor, etc.)
- The logical setting of a switch (on/off, true/false)
- The selection of one of a number of options (from a pick list or one out of a series of 'radio buttons' in a dialogue box)

Many different types of system require configuration parameters to be set, including ERP systems, LIMS systems, Distributed Control Systems, etc. Such systems are diverse in the way specific functions will be performed and the setting of the configuration parameters will determine exactly how the software module will function. Examples of the changes a configuration switch could make include:

- Whether or not a control loop is forward or reverse acting (positive or negative gain).

- Whether or not a Purchase Order requires one or two signatures and the value of purchase order for which a second approval signature will be required.
- Whether or not data from a sample can be saved with or without a supervisor's signature being required.

Once User Requirements and Functional Requirements have been determined and documented (in the User Requirements Specification and Functional Specification) the configuration settings need to be determined and documented in the Package Configuration Specification. There should also be clear traceability between the individual setting and the corresponding Functional and/or User Requirement.

A large or complex system may contain tens or hundreds of different modules, each of which may be of different GxP Criticality and a consistent method of determining the appropriate level of verification and/or testing should be defined and justified. This can serve to focus the verification/testing on the modules of medium or high GxP Criticality while reducing the overall level of testing.

Depending upon the GxP Criticality of the system, module or function the Package Configuration then needs to be verified and/or tested.

### 12.3 Verifying the Package Configuration

Verifying the Package Configuration is simply confirming that the configuration settings have been made as specified in the Package Configuration. This may be accomplished in a number of ways, dependent upon the GxP Criticality:

- For systems or functions that are not GxP critical it is acceptable for the person configuring the system to confirm the correct setting of the configuration parameters by completing a simple checklist (tick-boxes, with a single confirmation signature at the bottom).
- The package may be configured as defined in the Package Configuration and the person configuring the system is required to confirm each step either by signature or, preferably, by recording the actual configuration setting made. Since there is no independent verification of the Package Configuration this is only suitable for packages, applications or modules that have a low GxP Criticality. This would only be acceptable where an independent test of the Package Configuration is to follow, and where there is a high likelihood that any errors in the configuration would be detected in the subsequent testing.
- The package may be configured as defined in the Package Configuration and the person configuring the system is required to document each step by taking screen shots and by signing and dating them (as required for other test evidence).
- The package may be configured as defined in the Package Configuration and a witness independently records the configuration settings at the time they are made.
- After the system is configured an independent reviewer checks the system configuration settings against the Package Configuration Specification. Proof of such a review would be required, such as the completion of a summary sheet designed for the purpose. Dates and signatures should be recorded for either method.

These last three methods are suitable for verifying the configuration of systems or functions of medium or high GxP Criticality.

Any person involved in setting the configuration parameters should do so with a copy of the approved Package Configuration Specification in front of them. Anyone making, witnessing or reviewing such settings should also be sufficiently familiar with the package, application or module so that they can easily interpret the settings documented in the Package Configuration Specification and can tell when any errors are made.

For packages or modules that are not GxP Critical (or of low GxP Criticality) configuration verification is still a cost effective activity due to the reduction in subsequent errors that arise when a system is incorrectly configured.

For simple systems that are widely used in the Healthcare Industries, which have few configuration settings and where the GxP Criticality is low, it may not be necessary to conduct any further testing although this decision would need to be documented and justified. Similarly, where the use of a system and the resultant configuration settings are identical to other systems that the organisation has formally tested before it may be sufficient to just verify the configuration settings.

## 12.4 Functional Testing of the Package Configuration

As stated above, the configuration of a software module determines the exact way in which it will function. Verifying the correct configuration is a useful and worthwhile exercise but verification alone will only confirm that the settings have been made correctly and does not prove that the system functions in accordance with the System Requirements. For most applications this will still need to be formally tested.

In many cases it will be adequate to perform simple Functional Testing (i.e. to prove that the system meets the Users and Functional Requirements and functions as specified) and not to stress test the system (see Section 12.5).

This is justifiable in cases where:

- The package is a relatively simple one (with limited variation in functionality) and in widespread use in the regulated Healthcare Industries.
- The package is functionally identical to a system that has already been 'stress tested' (and the configuration has been verified as such).
- The GxP Criticality is low.

Such Functional Testing is conducted as part of the Software Integration Testing or System Acceptance Testing and would not require additional Package Configuration Testing.

## 12.5 Stress Testing of the Package Configuration

In some systems it will be necessary to not only functionally test the configuration of the system (to prove that it performs as specified during normal operations) but also to 'stress test' the system in order to determine the effects of abnormal operations.

This may be required where:

- The system is large or complex
- The package, application or module is not in common use in the Healthcare Industries (or this is the first time a particular organisation has used the package)
- The system is of medium or high GxP Criticality

In such cases the purpose of this additional testing is to demonstrate how the system will handle errors, incorrect attempts at operation or illegal operations.

Examples of such stress testing may include:

- Attempting to enter 'illegal' configuration settings and conflicting combinations in order to determine the effects of such settings (systems should, of course, reject illegal settings when attempts are made to enter them).
- Deliberately attempting to operate the system incorrectly, typically by attempting to perform GxP critical functions when logged in as a user with insufficient privileges (so called 'user profile testing').
- Attempting to deviate from the normal operational sequence when logged in as a privileged user, in order to confirm that the system correctly handles errors and/or enforces the correct sequence of operations (a requirement of 21 CFR Part 11).

Such stress testing can be conducted either as part of the Software Integration Testing or, perhaps more usefully, as a set of specific Package Configuration Tests conducted prior to the Software Integration Testing.

## 12.6 Configuration Settings in 'Non-Configurable' Systems

Even systems that are 'non-configurable' (i.e. the function is fixed, as in the case of software Category 2 or 3 or the function is determined solely by coding, as in the case of software category 5) may still have a number of configuration settings. These may typically be made at the operating system or database level and can impact on the security of the system, the integrity of the data, etc. Typically these configuration settings are used to control security on folders, the enabling of audit trails, etc.

Where they have a direct impact on product quality or data integrity, they should be defined as part of a Package Configuration Specification, which may be combined with a more general Software Design Specification. As a minimum, the setting of these should be verified as part of the system Installation Qualification and subject to formal change control.

CHAPTER 13

# Appendix C – Software Module Test Specifications and Testing

## 13.1 Defining the Software Module Test Strategy

Software Module Testing is required for all systems that include software that has been customised.

Where the entire system has been developed as a one-off solution, all of the software modules will require detailed Software Module Testing. In the case of a system which has limited customisation, only those software modules that are new or have been modified need to be subject to Software Module Testing.

Software modules that have been formally tested previously need not be subject to Software Module Testing on a project so long as:

- The supplier (or possibly the user) can reference the previous test results.
- The software module has been under formal change control as part of a recognised quality system and is demonstrably the same version.
- No other changes in the system (such as the hardware, application version, database version, operating system version, etc.) invalidate the previous testing.

The Test Strategy should clearly identify which software modules are subject to Software Module Testing, which are excluded and the rationale for this.

The objectives of the Software Module Tests should be clearly traceable to the appropriate sections of the Software Module Design Specification(s). Meeting the objectives of the Software Module Test Scripts should clearly demonstrate that the software is designed and operates as specified.

## 13.2 Examples of Software Modules

While a full definition of modular software is outside the scope of this guideline, examples could include:

- C/C++
- Visual Basic
- Ladder Logic
- Java Script
- DOS batch files

## 13.3 Stress (Challenge) Testing of Software Modules

Prior to testing, all software modules subject to testing should have undergone a formal source code review and should be under change control.

The nature and extent of the testing should be appropriate to the GxP Criticality of the specific module. Modules which are non GxP-critical should be subject to good testing practice and test results may be recorded by use of a simple checklist. Software modules that are GxP-critical require formal Test Scripts to be developed.

Modules with a low GxP criticality may be subject to Functional Testing within their normal operating range, with no requirement for stress testing on the basis that there is a good likelihood of any fault being discovered in a subsequent stage of testing.

Modules of medium and high GxP criticality should be subject to stress (or challenge) testing across a wide range of illegal or invalid inputs:

- Enter discrete inputs (illegal patterns such as device feedback signals from a valve or a motor indicating that a valve is both open and closed or that a motor is both running and stopped)
- Analogue inputs (above or below normal ranges)
- Operator inputs (out of range or illegal/random 'garbage' inputs)
- Illegal conditions (similar to discrete input patterns as above but with a wider range of input types simultaneously tested)

The degree to which the tests attempt to 'break' the module (i.e. cause the software to freeze, enter a recursive loop, cause a hardware or operating system error, cause unexpected or illegal output, etc.) should be applicable to the GxP criticality and complexity of the module. Modules that are too complex to test adequately should be deconstructed into a greater number of separate modules.

CHAPTER 14

# Appendix D – Software Integration Test Specifications and Testing

## 14.1 The Purpose and Scope of Software Integration Testing

The purpose of System Integration Testing is basically to ensure that the different components of a system or solution function correctly together. This may be where different applications are integrated into a single solution (for instance, a standard Laboratory Information System is integrated with a standard mail server to send e-mails or where a standard weighing and dispensing system is integrated into a standard ERP system). This is also required where customised GAMP category 5 software is included as part of a solution.

Where the solution is mature, properly developed and well proven in the market place and the user has taken appropriate steps to confirm this, there is usually no need to conduct System Integration Testing; System Acceptance Testing alone will suffice. However, System Integration Testing will be required when:

- The system is a complex one, consisting of many software components and it is not a mature product, well proven in the market place.
- Any existing module is customised in any way. Its interfacing and integrating with other modules must be tested but the extent of such testing may be limited to the interfaces with the customised software. Note that this may also include the reconfiguration of GAMP category 4 software (Package Configuration) where the new configuration is significantly different from that which is commonly used in the industry.
- Any new functionality is developed within a system.

Prior to System Integration Testing the individual applications or modules will have either been defined as mature and standard in the market place or will have been subjected to Software Module Testing at an appropriate level. The purpose of Software Integration Testing is, therefore, to ensure that the various software components all function correctly together.

At a higher level, Software Integration Testing is also used to test the interfaces between different systems. In order to evaluate the functioning of the interface it is necessary that the individual systems (or at least those functions in the system responsible for handling the interface) have been fully tested.

When defining Software Integration Tests the purpose is not to challenge test the individual modules or systems, but to ensure that the modules or systems function correctly together in a robust, reliable and predictable manner. Where appropriate, stress testing (or challenge testing) may be part of this.

The objectives of the Software Integration Tests should be clearly traceable to the appropriate sections of the Software Design Specification(s). Meeting the objectives of the Software Design

Test Scripts should clearly demonstrate that the overall system is designed and operates as specified.

### 14.2 System Integration Tests

When designing appropriate tests the following questions should be asked:

- What would happen if one of the modules or systems stopped responding or functioned in an abnormal manner? Would the integrated modules or systems also stop functioning?
- What would happen if the modules or systems become unsynchronised? Are all messages appropriately identified to allow responses to be correctly attributed to queries? Is there sufficient buffer capacity to store queries whilst waiting for outstanding responses?
- Is the system infrastructure capable of handling the anticipated traffic? This may apply to network components as well as the data bus in an embedded system?
- Can the system detect data that has been corrupted by, or between, different software modules or components? The ability of individual modules to reject out of range or corrupt data should have been checked at the software module level, but this is worth checking for critical functions.
- Are there incompatibilities in data formats? This may apply to numerical formats (such as the length of integer words or floating point numbers) or encoding standards, such as binary coded decimal.
- What would happen if a software module, component or device would not relinquish control of a network or carried on transmitting continuously? What effect would this have on network traffic and system performance?
- Are appropriate checks on the validity of originating modules or devices made? Would it be possible for another device or component to be attached to the system and would this be detected?
- What would happen if the user of one system attempted to gain access to a different system? Are the user profiles recognised by all components in the system? Are users with inappropriate levels of access rejected by all modules and functions? This is especially pertinent if the application is reliant upon user authentication at the operating system or network level.

Such questions help to determine the nature of the System Integration Tests and also how challenging such tests should be. Performing a risk analysis will help to determine where the critical risks lie and where test effort should be focused.

CHAPTER 15

# Appendix E – System Acceptance Test Specifications and Testing

## 15.1 The Purpose of System Acceptance Testing

All challenge testing should have been conducted as part of the previous levels of testing. The purpose of System Acceptance Testing is to demonstrate that the system functions in accordance with the requirements of the Functional Specification. This basically means that it functions how it was designed to perform.

As part of this, some of the User Requirements may be tested as well (it does what it is supposed to do) and System Acceptance Tests can form part of both the Operational Qualification and the Performance Qualification.

System Acceptance Testing usually has some contractual significance and is usually witnessed by the user. Sign off of the System Acceptance Tests is usually defined as a milestone in the project and may well be the point at which the system is handed over to the user.

## 15.2 The Nature of System Acceptance Testing

System acceptance testing is functional in nature. System Acceptance Tests are usually designed around the normal functioning of the system and serve to demonstrate that the system functions as specified in the Functional Specification. Part of the tests may be conducted as part of the Factory Acceptance Tests and may be completed as part of the Site Acceptance Tests.

Normal operation and work flow will be demonstrated. This may be picking and stacking pallets, the raising of a purchase order, the approval of a CAD drawing and so on. These functions will be tested or witnessed by the actual users of the system (profile challenge testing, to demonstrate that other users are not able to perform these tasks is conducted prior to the System Acceptance Tests).

The objectives of the System Acceptance Tests should be clearly traceable to the appropriate sections of the Functional Specification and possibly to the User Requirements Specification. Meeting the objectives of the System Acceptance Test Scripts should clearly demonstrate that the system is functioning as specified.

## 15.3 Establishing a Performance Monitoring Baseline

The test results taken during the System Acceptance Tests can be used to establish a baseline for the future performance monitoring of the system. When the system is first installed the operation of the system should be at its peak (hard discs are relatively empty, network traffic should be within design limits, overheating should not be a problem and system grounding and earthing should be optimum).

This may degrade over time, but unless a suitable set of baseline test data are established, it will be impossible to make any meaningful comparisons. Although not formally part of the System Acceptance tests (unless certain criteria are included in the User Requirements or Functional Specification) it is nevertheless useful to include such testing.

This may be conducted during the Performance Qualification phase of the system testing, where reliable data can be established over an appropriate time scale.

CHAPTER 16

# Appendix F – Risk-Based Testing

GxP Priority is just one risk factor to consider when determining the degree of risk associated with a particular software module, application or function.

For instance, a software module may be of high GxP criticality but if it has been tested by the supplier, used by hundreds of other pharmaceutical companies and has not been modified, the risk of using such a module may be low and it may require little or no testing.

On the other hand a software module may have been customised by a development team working under extreme time constraints, with no prior experience of conducting source code review, with no coding standards, using a language which is relatively new to the market and which they have never used before. If this module is of medium GxP Priority, does it really require less testing that the module of high GxP criticality?

The test strategy must therefore take a number of factors into account and these can be given a weighting factor. GxP Criticality and GAMP software and hardware categories are just two factors that may be taken into consideration. The overall risk can then be calculated and used in the development of an appropriate testing strategy.

The table below provides an example of such a weighting, with various risk factors included. This is obviously a more complex approach than one solely based upon GxP Criticality and software/hardware category and may only be applicable to large organisations involved in testing a wide range of systems on a more-or-less continuous basis. If organisations decide to use such an approach they may wish to discuss and agree risk factors, categories and weightings appropriate to their own organisation (Table 16.1).

The different system components can be assessed against the risk factors and categories above and a scoring given based on the sum of the weighting factors. Different modules can then be assigned the different test approaches.

As an example, if the above weightings were used, the maximum score would be 100. For software this may equate to (Table 16.2).

**Table 16.1 – Example of System Risk Factors**

| | | | | | |
|---|---|---|---|---|---|
| Risk Factor | GAMP Software Category | | | | |
| Category | 1 | 2 | 3 | 4 | 5 |
| Weighting | 0 | 1 | 3 | 5 | 10 |
| Risk Factor | GAMP Hardware Category | | | | |
| Category | 1 | 2 | | | |
| Weighting | 0 | 10 | | | |
| Risk Factor | GxP Priority | | | | |
| Category | Low | | Medium | | High |
| Weighting | 5 | | 10 | | 20 |
| Risk Factor | Business Criticality | | | | |
| Category | Low | | Medium | | High |
| Weighting | 5 | | 10 | | 20 |
| Risk Factor | Software Module Complexity | | | | |
| Category | Low | | Medium | | High |
| Weighting | 1 | | 3 | | 5 |
| Risk Factor | Established History of Module/Application | | | | |
| Category | Mature | | Established | | New |
| Weighting | 1 | | 3 | | 5 |
| Risk Factor | Speed of Development | | | | |
| Category | Slow | | Normal | | Fast |
| Weighting | 5 | | 3 | | 10 |
| Risk Factor | Supplier Track Record | | | | |
| Category | Excellent | Good | Average | Poor | None |
| Weighting | 0 | 3 | 5 | 7 | 10 |
| Risk Factor | History of Development Tools | | | | |
| Category | Excellent | Good | Average | Poor | New |
| Weighting | 1 | 2 | 3 | 5 | 5 |
| Risk Factor | Size of Development Team | | | | |
| Category | 1 | 2 | 3–4 | 5–9 | 10+ |
| Weighting | 3 | 1 | 3 | 4 | 5 |

**Table 16.2 – Example of Test Approaches Based Upon Risk Factors**

| *Rating* | *Test Approach* |
|---|---|
| 1 to 10 | No specific testing required. Will be tested as part of overall System Acceptance Testing (Functional Testing).<br>25% of System Acceptance Test Specification and Results are subject to Quality function review and approval. |
| 11 to 20 | Will be tested as part of overall System Acceptance Testing (Functional Testing). Testing outside standard operating ranges is required in order to predict failure modes.<br>100% of System Acceptance Test Specification and Results are subject to Quality function review and approval. |
| 20 to 35 | In additional to System Acceptance (Functional) Testing, the system must be subjected to stress testing during normal operating conditions to challenge:<br>– Basic system (log-in) access<br>– User (role) specific functional access<br>– System administration access<br>– Network security<br>50% of Package Configuration Test Specifications and 50% of related Results are subject to independent Quality function review and approval.<br>100% of all System Acceptance Test Specifications and Results are subject to independent Quality function review and approval. |
| 36 to 50 | In additional to System Acceptance (Functional) Testing, the system must be subjected to comprehensive stress testing across normal and abnormal operating conditions in order to challenge:<br>– Basic system (log-in) access<br>– User (role) specific functional access<br>– System administration access<br>– Network security<br>100% of Package Configuration Test Specifications and 100% of related Results are subject to independent Quality function review.<br>100% of all System Acceptance Test Specifications and Results are subject to independent Quality function review. |
| 51 to 65 | Software Module Testing mandated prior to System Integration Tests and System Acceptance Testing.<br>Only testing within standard operating range required<br>25% of Software Module Test Specifications and 10% of all Software Module Test Results are subject to independent Quality function review.<br>25% of all Software Integration Specification and related test Results subject to independent Quality function review.<br>100% of all System Acceptance Test Specifications and Results are subject to independent Quality function review. |
| 66 to 80 | Software Module Testing mandated prior to System Integration Tests and System Acceptance Testing.<br>Testing only within standard operating range required for Software Module Tests.<br>Testing outside standard operating range required for Software Integration Tests in order to predict failure modes.<br>50% of Software Module Test Specifications and 50% of all Software Module Test Results are subject to independent Quality function review. |
| 66 to 80 | 50% of all Software Integration Specification and related test Results are subject to independent Quality function review.<br>100% of all System Acceptance Test Specifications and Results are subject to independent Quality function review. |
| 81 to 100 | Software Module Testing mandated prior to System Integration Tests and System Acceptance Testing.<br>Testing only within standard operating range required for Software Module Tests.<br>Testing outside standard operating range required for Software Integration Tests in order to predict failure modes.<br>100% of Software Module Test Specifications and 100% of all Software Module Test Results are subject to independent Quality function review.<br>25% of all Software Integration Specification and related test Results are subject to independent Quality function review.<br>100% of all System Acceptance Test Specifications and Results are subject to independent Quality function review. |

CHAPTER 17

# Appendix G – Traceability Matrices

The following tables summarise the traceability between the various activities and deliverables associated with the development of Test Specifications and the associated testing. It should be noted that the actual interrelationship of these would usually be defined in the overall Validation Plan.

For each of the tables, input activities are listed on the left. Dependant activities to which they may have an input are listed along the top of the table. This means activities across to the top are traceable to activities down the left hand side only when there is a tick (√) in the intersecting cell.

## 17.1 The Development of the Test Specifications

**Table 17.1 – Test Specifications Traceability**

| *Activities along the top are traceable to activities listed below* | *Hardware Test Specification* | *Software Module Test Specification* | *Package Configuration Test Specification* | *Software Integration Test Specification* | *System Acceptance Test Specification* |
|---|---|---|---|---|---|
| Validation Plan | √ | √ | √ | √ | √ |
| Project Quality Plan | √ | √ | √ | √ | √ |
| Test Strategy | √ | √ | √ | √ | √ |
| Hardware Specification | √ | | | | |
| Software Module Specification(s) | | √ | | | |
| Package Configuration Specification | | | √ | | |
| Software Design Specification | | | | √ | |
| Functional Specification | | | | | √ |

## 17.2 The Development of the Test Scripts

**Table 17.2 – Test Script Traceability**

| *Activities along the top are traceable to activities listed below* | *Hardware Test Scripts* | *Software Module Test Scripts* | *Package Configuration Test Scripts* | *Software Integration Test Scripts* | *System Acceptance Test Scripts* |
|---|---|---|---|---|---|
| Validation Plan | √ | √ | √ | √ | √ |
| Project Quality Plan | √ | √ | √ | √ | √ |
| Test Strategy | √ | √ | √ | √ | √ |
| Hardware Test Specification | √ | | | | |
| Applicable section of Hardware Specification | √ | | | | |
| Software Module Test Specification | | √ | | | |
| Applicable section of Software Module Specification(s) | | √ | | | |
| Package Configuration Test Specification | | | √ | | |
| Applicable section of Package Configuration Specification | | | √ | | |
| Software Integration Test Specification | | | | √ | |
| Applicable section of Software Design Specification | | | | √ | |
| System Acceptance Test Specification | | | | | √ |
| Applicable section of Functional Specification | | | | | √ |

## 17.3 Test Execution

**Table 17.3 – Test Execution Traceability**

| *Activities along the top are traceable to activities listed below* | *Hardware Testing* | *Software Module Testing* | *Package Configuration Testing* | *Software Integration Testing* | *System Acceptance Testing* |
|---|---|---|---|---|---|
| Validation Plan | √ | √ | √ | √ | √ |
| Project Quality Plan | √ | √ | √ | √ | √ |
| Test Strategy | √ | √ | √ | √ | √ |
| Hardware Specification, Test Specification and Test Scripts | √ | | | | |
| Tested Hardware | | | | | √ |
| Software Module Specification, Test Specification and Test Scripts | | √ | | | |
| Tested Software Modules | | | | √ | √ |
| Package Configuration Specification, Test Specification and Test Scripts Tested Package Configuration | | | √ | | |
| Software Design Specification, Integration Test Specification and Test Scripts | | | | | |

## 17.4 Test Reporting and Qualification

**Table 17.4 – Test Reporting Traceability**

| *Activities along the top are traceable to activities listed below* | *Hardware Test Report* | *Software Module Test Report* | *Package Configuration Test Report* | *Software Integration Test Report* | *System Acceptance Test Report* | *Overall System Test Report* | *Installation Qualification* | *Operational Qualification* | *Performance Qualification* | *Validation Report* |
|---|---|---|---|---|---|---|---|---|---|---|
| Hardware Test Results | √ | | | | | | √ | | | |
| Tested Hardware | | | | | | | √ | | | |
| Hardware Test Report | | | | | | | √ | | | |
| Software Module Test Results | | √ | | | | | | √ | | |
| Tested Software Modules | | | | | | | | √ | | |
| Software Module Test Report | | | | | | | | √ | | |
| Package Configuration Test Results | | | √ | | | | | √ | √ | |
| Tested Package Configuration | | | | | | | | √ | √ | |
| Package Configuration Test Report | | | | | | | | √ | √ | |
| Software Integration Test Results | | | | √ | | | | √ | √ | |
| Software Integration Test Report | | | | | | | | √ | √ | |
| System Acceptance Test Results | | | | | √ | | | √ | √ | |
| System Acceptance Test Report | | | | | | | | √ | √ | |
| Overall System Test Report | | | | | | | | √ | √ | √ |
| Tested System | | | | | | | | √ | √ | √ |

CHAPTER 18

# Appendix H – Test Script Templates

The following example provides details of a Test Script Template and can be used as the basis for developing project specific versions. An example sheet is also included.

## 18.1 Basic Template for a Test Script

Note that fields to be completed during the actual test or as part of the acceptance are shaded.

| | |
|---|---|
| **System Acceptance Test Specification**<br>**Individual System Acceptance Test Record Sheet** | |
| **Project No:**<br>**Project Name:**<br>**Test Reference:**<br>**System Function under test:** | |
| **Functional Description of System Function under test:** | |
| **Specific Test Prerequisites (not included in General Section)** | |
| **Specific Test Method:** | |
| **Description of Test:** | |
| **Test Methods to be used:** | |
| **Detailed Instructions:** | |

Page 1 of 2

| **System Acceptance Test Specification**<br>**Individual System Acceptance Test Record Sheet** | |
|---|---|
| **Project No:** | |
| **Project Name:** | |
| **Test Reference:** | |
| **System Function under test:** | |

| **Input** | **Expected Result** | **Unacceptable Result** | **Actual Result** |
|---|---|---|---|
| | | | |
| | | | |
| **Maximum number of Repeat Tests:** | | | |
| **Test Run Number:** | | | |
| **Test Result (tick ONE box below):** | | | |
| **Pass:** ☐ | | **Fail:** ☐ | |
| **Reset/Further Actions:** | | | |
| **Test conducted by:** | | | |
| **(Print Name):** | | | |
| **Date:** | | | |
| **Test Reviewed/Accepted by:** | | | |
| **(Print Name):** | | | |
| **Date:** | | | |

## 18.2 Example of a Specific Test Script

Note that this Test Script does not contain detailed instructions and references a test method. Fields to be completed during the actual test or as part of the acceptance are shaded.

**System Acceptance Test Specification**
**Individual System Acceptance Test Record Sheet**

| | |
|---|---|
| **Project No:** | AC95003 |
| **Project Name:** | Acme Pharmaceuticals Building 30 |
| **Test Reference:** | CFG 034 (Revision 1.02) |
| **System Function under test:** | Centrifuge Operation |

**Functional Description of System Function under test:**
The system will automatically increase the speed of the centrifuge, from rest to a minimum speed of 3,000 rpm over a period of between 1 minute 30 seconds and 2 minutes. The centrifuge will run at a minimum speed of 3,000 rpm for a period not less than two minutes and not exceeding 2 minutes fifteen seconds. The centrifuge shall then decelerate, achieving rest in not more than 30 seconds.

Page 1 of 4

**Specific Test Prerequisites (not included in General Section)**
None

**Specific Test Method:**
Equipment Module Test – See General Section, 1.2.4.

**Description of Test:**
The selected equipment module (Centrifuge 034) will be placed in manual mode and the status set to 'manual default'. The operation of the centrifuge connected to the test system will then be observed.

**Test Methods to be used:**
The test will be initiated via manual entry of data into the control faceplate for Centrifuge 034. The operation of the Centrifuge will then be observed.

**Detailed Instructions:**

1. Select the faceplate for Centrifuge 034. If not already in 'MAN' mode, select 'MAN' mode.
2. Set the Status of Centrifuge 034 to 'run' (entering the Engineers password when prompted).
3. Observe and note the time taken to reach full running speed, the time at full speed and the time to decelerate. Note the speed reached (displayed on the centrifuge local display) at the end of the run up period and the lowest speed observed during the run.
4. Record the observed values displayed as the 'comparison data' value.
5. Select the control faceplate for Centrifuge 034. Select 'AUTO' mode.

Page 2 of 4

| | |
|---|---|
| **System Acceptance Test Specification**<br>**Individual System Acceptance Test Record Sheet** | |
| **Project No:** | AC95003 |
| **Project Name:** | Acme Pharmaceuticals Building 30 |
| **Test Reference:** | CFG 034 (Revision 1.02) |
| **Software Module under test:** | Centrifuge Operation |

| **Input** | **Expected Result** | **Unacceptable Result** | **Actual Result** |
|---|---|---|---|
| **Run up time** | >1m30s, < 2m00s | <1m30s, > 2m00s | |
| **Speed reached** | 3000 rpm +/– 50 | <2950, > 3050 | |
| **Run time** | >2m00s, < 2m15s | <2m00s, > 2m15s | |
| **Minimum run speed** | 2950 rpm | < 2950rpm | |
| **Deceleration time** | < 30s | > 30s | |
| **Maximum number of Repeat Tests:** | | 1 | |
| **Test Run Number:** | | | |
| **Test Result (tick ONE box below):** | | | |
| **Pass:** ☐ | | **Fail:** ☐ | |

Page 3 of 4

| | |
|---|---|
| **Reset/Further Actions:** | |
| **Test conducted by:** | |
| **(Print Name):** | |
| **Date:** | |
| **Test Reviewed/Accepted by:** | |
| **(Print Name):** | |
| **Date:** | |

Page 4 of 4

## 18.3 Example of a Test Script with Detailed Instructions

The following test script provides detailed instructions for each step (in this case, for testing an ERP system).

Integration Test Scenario <Test Scenario Reference>

This is a GxP Critical Test and the following test controls MUST be applied:

### Pass Criteria

In order for a Process Step to pass the test, the following criteria must be fulfilled:

- All test prerequisites and conditions must have been set-up prior to test execution.
- All Test Scripts associated with the Process Step must have been successfully executed, with test evidence provided as described below
- The tester shall sign off each Test Script, to confirm that the Test Script was executed as documented, that the actual results matched the expected results, that the test acceptance criteria were met and that there were no test anomalies.

In order for a Business Requirement to pass the test the following criteria must be fulfilled:

- All of the Process Steps associated with the Business Requirement shall have passed as defined above and shall have been reviewed by the Test Stream Leader and the implementation stream Validation Consultant.
- All test incidents shall have been resolved.
- The Business Process Test Review Section shall be signed by the Test Stream Leader and the implementation stream Validation Consultant.

### Test Evidence

Evidence shall be provided to demonstrate the successful execution of each individual test script. Evidence is not required for each step. Evidence shall be provided either by:

- Attaching a screen shot of the test outcome to the executed Test Script, which clearly demonstrates that the acceptance criteria has been achieved. Attachments shall be signed and dated by the Tester OR
- A witness shall observe the execution of the entire Test Script, and shall sign and date the witness section of the Test Script sign-off.

| | | | |
|---|---|---|---|
| SCENARIO: | Quality Inspection in Production <Test Scenario Reference> | OWNER: | <Mi Services> |
| BUSINESS CASE: | Production Order with Quality Inspection using Inspection Points | STATUS: | <Draft> |
| DESCRIPTION: | Recording Quality Results for Inspection Point Processing | RUN NO.: | |
| ACCEPTANCE CRITERIA: | <Acceptance Criteria for Test> | RUN DATE: | |

**SETUP DATA**

| DATA OBJECT | VALUE/CODE | DESCRIPTION | COMMENTS AND NOTES |
|---|---|---|---|
| Company Code | | | |
| Plant | | | |
| Storage Location | | | |
| Material Master | | | **Inspection type 03** |
| Routing/Ref. Op. Set | | | |
| Test Data Set (where used) | <reference> version (N.n) | | |

**NOTES and INSTRUCTIONS**

1. Run number and date shall be entered at the top right of this page for every test.
2. Expected results reference set-up data unless otherwise stated.
3. GxP Code identifies 21CFR Part 11 requirements in accordance with the specified Predicate Rules.

| | | | |
|---|---|---|---|
| **'R =':** | **Records required by the applicable Predicate Rules** | **E:** | **Record is stored electronically** |
| **'r =':** | **Record required for other business purposes (default)** | **M:** | **Manual (paper record) is stored** |
| ***'S =':*** | ***Signature required by the applicable Predicate Rules*** | **0:** | **No record is stored (required)** |
| ***'s =':*** | ***Signature required for other business purposes (default)*** | ***E:*** | ***Signature is applied electronically*** |
| | | ***M:*** | ***Hand-written signature is applied (usually to a paper record)*** |
| | | ***0:*** | ***No signature is used*** |

4. User Profile identifies User Profile used for testing
5. Tester name must be entered in full for each step where the main Tester is not conducting the transaction test. The main Tester should initial each step.
6. 'Pass' or 'Fail' must be entered in full for each step.
7. Comment references should be recorded in the final column for all comments added on the final sheet. Where applicable, comments shall be used to record details of any attachments.

TRANSACTIONAL STEPS – < Test Scenario Reference> <Run Number> < Run Date>

| No | BUSINESS PROCESS STEPS/BPP NUMBER | TRANS. CODE | INPUT DATA/ SPECIAL INFORMATION | EXPECTED RESULT | GxP CODE | USER PROFILE | TESTER NAME or INITIALS | RESULT | COMMENT REF |
|---|---|---|---|---|---|---|---|---|---|
| 0 | Release production order. | CO02 | Production Order Number. | Order status changed to 'Released'. Inspection Lot created. | | | | | |
| 1 | Review Inspection Lot created as a result of the release of the production order. | QA03 | Material or Production order number | Inspection lot number | | | | | |
| 2 | Results recording for an inspection point for characteristics or specifications for the inspection lot. | QE11 or QE51 or QE712 | Inspection lot number operation, and inspection point identification. | Results will be evaluated as accept or reject according to the data recorded for the characteristics or specifications for each inspection point. Also a confirmation will be posted to the production order. | | | | | |
| 3 | Defects recording for characteristics/ specifications. | QE11 or QE51 or QE71 | Inspection lot number, operation and inspection point identification. | | | | | | |
| 4 | Usage decision for the inspection lot. | QA11 or QVM3 | Inspection lot number. | Usage Decision made. | | | | | |

| Comments: <Test Scenario Reference> <Run Number> < Run Date> | |
|---|---|
| Number | Comment |
| | |
| | |
| | |
| | |
| | |

PASS/FAIL (Delete as appropriate)

Signed (Tester) Date (dd-mm-yy)

Witnessed (if required) Date (dd-mm-yy)

CHAPTER 19

# Appendix I – Checklists

The following checklists provide a list of useful questions to ask when preparing a System Test Specification. By answering these questions the author of such a document will be able to determine whether or not the System Test Specification can usefully be started and completed and whether or not the actual System Acceptance Tests can be conducted.

Note that the some of the questions and answers will be specific to the type of Test Specification being developed (Hardware, Software Module, Package Configuration, System Integration or System Acceptance). Only when all the answers in a particular section have been answered should the relevant work commence.

## 19.1 Checklist 1

**Before Starting the Test Specification**

| **Question** | **Answer** |
| --- | --- |
| **Validation Plan/Project Quality Plan** | |
| Is the Validation Plan/Project Quality Plan available? | **Yes/No** |
| • If it is, is it signed-off and released? | **Yes/No** |
| Is the Validation Plan/Project Quality Plan clear in specifying a need for this Test Specification? | **Yes/No** |
| • If it states that one is not required, does the supplier's own Project Quality Plan require one? | **Yes/No** |
| Does the Validation Plan/Project Quality Plan allow this Test Specification to be combined with any other document? | **Yes/No** |
| • If it does, which other documents? | |
| Does the Validation Plan/Project Quality Plan place specific requirements on the supplier for reviewing this Test Specification? | **Yes/No** |
| • If not, what requirements are there in the supplier's own Project Quality Plan? | |
| Does the Validation Plan/Project Quality Plan require the user to review and accept this Test Specification? | **Yes/No** |

| Question | Answer |
|---|---|
| **Test Strategy** | |
| Is the Test Strategy | |
| • An integral part of the Validation Plan? | **Yes/No** |
| • An integral part of the Project Quality Plan? | **Yes/No** |
| • An integral part of a Qualification Protocol? | **Yes/No** |
| • A separate document? | **Yes/No** |
| Is there a separate Test Strategy Document detailing | |
| • The testing rationale? | **Yes/No** |
| • The relationship between the various types and phases of testing? | **Yes/No** |
| • The relationship between the supplier's FAT, SAT and the IQ, OQ and PQ? | **Yes/No** |
| **Specification** | |
| Is the Appropriate Specification available (Functional, Hardware, Software, Package Configuration or Software Module)? | **Yes/No** |
| • If it is, is it signed-off and released? | **Yes/No** |
| How does the Specification impact or influence the System Acceptance Test Specification? | |

## 19.2 Checklist 2

**The Development of the Test Specification**

| Question | Answer |
|---|---|
| Does the title block of the document include: | |
| • The project name? | **Yes/No** |
| • The document title? | **Yes/No** |
| • An up-to-date revision number (subject to proper change control)? | **Yes/No** |
| • Details of the author(s)? | **Yes/No** |
| • Space for approval signatures? | **Yes/No** |
| Are details of the document QA process referred to in the document? | **Yes/No** |
| Is the scope of the document clearly defined, including: | |
| • The relationship with other validation life cycle documents? | **Yes/No** |
| • The reasons for the grouping and ordering of tests? | **Yes/No** |
| • Details of functions not tested and why? | **Yes/No** |
| • Allowable deviations from general test methodology? | **Yes/No** |
| Has a glossary been included or referenced? | **Yes/No** |
| Are general principles and test methodology clearly explained, including: | |
| • The principles of testing? | **Yes/No** |
| • Standard test methods? | **Yes/No** |

- How results should be recorded? **Yes/No**
- How tests are 'signed-off' and accepted? **Yes/No**

Is sufficient detail included or referenced for all of the above? **Yes/No**

Are general test prerequisites clearly explained, including:

- Required system hardware and software? **Yes/No**
- Required test equipment? **Yes/No**
- Required test software? **Yes/No**
- Required test datasets? **Yes/No**
- Required process, plant or equipment? **Yes/No**
- Required test documentation? **Yes/No**
- Prior tests? **Yes/No**
- Is sufficient detail included or referenced for all of the above? **Yes/No**

## 19.3 Checklist 3

**Before starting any Test Script**

**Question** **Answer**

**Validation Plan/Project Quality Plan/Test Strategy**

Is the Validation Plan/Project Quality Plan/Test Strategy available? **Yes/No**

- If it is, is it signed-off and released? **Yes/No**

Does the Validation Plan/Project Quality Plan/Test Strategy provide sufficient details about the format and quality of the Test Scripts? **Yes/No**

Does the Validation Master Plan/Project Quality Plan/Test Strategy specify who will be required to 'sign-off' the Test Scripts? **Yes/No**

Does the Validation Plan/Project Quality Plan/Test Strategy specify whether or not the user will be required to approve individual Test Scripts? **Yes/No**

Does the Validation Plan/Project Quality Plan/Test Strategy specify whether or not a user review of the Test Scripts will be part of the Operational Qualification or not? **Yes/No**

**Functional/Design Specification**

Is the appropriate Functional/Design Specification available? **Yes/No**

- If it is, is it signed-off and released? **Yes/No**

How do the individual sections of the Functional/Design Specification impact or influence the individual Test Scripts?

**Test Specification**

**Is the appropriate Test Specification complete?** **Yes/No**

How much detail is included in the Test Specification and how much is required to be written in the Individual Test Scripts? Is there any gap or overlap?

## 19.4 Checklist 4

| **The Development of the Individual Test Scripts**<br>**Question** | **Answer** |
|---|---|
| Does each test have: | |
| • A unique test reference? | **Yes/No** |
| • A test name? | **Yes/No** |
| • Details of, or reference to, a complete functional description of the test item? | **Yes/No** |
| Are specific test prerequisites clearly explained, including: | |
| • Required system hardware and software? | **Yes/No** |
| • Required test equipment? | **Yes/No** |
| • Required test software? | **Yes/No** |
| • Required test datasets? | **Yes/No** |
| • Required process, plant or equipment? | **Yes/No** |
| • Required test documentation? | **Yes/No** |
| • Prior tests? | **Yes/No** |
| Is sufficient detail included or referenced for all of the above where they differ from details in the General Section of the System Acceptance Test Specification? | **Yes/No** |
| Are specific principles and test methodology clearly explained, including: | |
| • A description of the test? | **Yes/No** |
| • Standard test methods? | **Yes/No** |
| • Expected results (pass/fail criteria)? | **Yes/No** |
| • How the test results are recorded? | **Yes/No** |
| • How tests are 'signed-off' and accepted? | **Yes/No** |
| • How and when tests are repeated? | **Yes/No** |
| • Reset actions? | **Yes/No** |
| • Setting up for subsequent tests? | **Yes/No** |
| Is sufficient detail included or referenced for all of the above where they differ from details in the Test Specification? | **Yes/No** |

## 19.5 Checklist 5

| **Before Conducting any System Acceptance Test**<br>**Question** | **Answer** |
|---|---|
| Is the full System Acceptance Test Specification to hand? | **Yes/No** |
| • If it is, is it signed-off and released? | **Yes/No** |

Is the relevant individual section of the System Acceptance Test Specification easily to hand? **Yes/No**

- If it is, is it signed-off and released? **Yes/No**

Is the relevant Test Record Sheet available and to hand? **Yes/No**

Are all the prerequisites items available and properly set up?

- Required system hardware and software? **Yes/No**
- Required test equipment? **Yes/No**
- Required test software? **Yes/No**
- Required test datasets? **Yes/No**
- Required process, plant or equipment? **Yes/No**
- Required test documentation? **Yes/No**
- Prior tests? **Yes/No**

Is any other necessary documentation to hand? **Yes/No**

Are the Test Engineer and Witness suitably qualified/trained/experienced to conduct and sign-off the test? **Yes/No**

## 19.6 Checklist 6

**Prior to Signing-Off a System Acceptance Test**

| Question | Answer |
|---|---|
| Were the step-by-step, documented instructions properly followed? | **Yes/No** |
| • Did this include set-up, prerequisites, testing and reset? | **Yes/No** |
| Was the Test Engineer suitably qualified/trained/experienced to conduct and sign-off the test? | **Yes/No** |
| Were the results as expected (as per documented acceptance criteria)? | **Yes/No** |
| Were the results properly recorded and documented? | **Yes/No** |
| Was the number of test failures within the allowable maximum? | **Yes/No** |
| Was the Test Script properly signed and dated by the Test Engineer? | **Yes/No** |

CHAPTER 20

# Appendix J – References and Acknowledgments

## 20.1 References


[1] Good Automated Manufacturing Practice (GAMP) Guide, version 4. Published by ISPE

[2] Guidance for Industry, 21 CFR Part 11; Electronic Records; Electronic Signatures – (draft guidance from the FDA, published February 2003)


## 20.2 Acknowledgments


From a personal perspective, my thanks go to Kevin Francis of Mercury Interactive and to Andrew Dickson of G4 Consulting for their insights into 'state-of-the-art' computerised test management tools.

To everyone at Mi Services Group; thanks for encouraging us all to get involved with defining industry best practice, and especially to Rachel and Nichola for correcting my grammar.

I should also mention all those colleagues who I have had the privilege (and sometimes the misfortune) to test with over the years. They are too numerous to mention, but in their own way they have all contributed to the development of this guide.

My special thanks go to Chris Reid of Integrity Solutions for his useful comments when originally editing this guideline, and to Tim Cronin at Fluor, for his constructive review comments — quite a task (how they found the time is quite beyond me).

Thanks are also due to Sue Horwood, who remains dedicated to the task of producing and publishing practical guidance for the industry at affordable prices.

And finally, from a personal perspective, to my family — for all their encouragement and patience and for sticking with this guide through its many incarnations.

Your support is all very much appreciated.

# Index